CW01161035

Me, my space, my place

To dear Par
with some fond memories
Maris

To Marjorie

Copyright 2009 by the author of this book Maris Cole. The book author retains sole copyright to the contributions to this book.

Published by The Play Close Press,
The Mead, Great Somerford, Chippenham, Wiltshire
SN15 5JB

Further copies of this publication can be obtained from:
www.blurb.com

ISBN 978-0-9561804-0-7

The Blurb-provided layout designs and graphic elements are copyright Blurb Inc., 2009. This book was created using the Blurb creative publishing service.

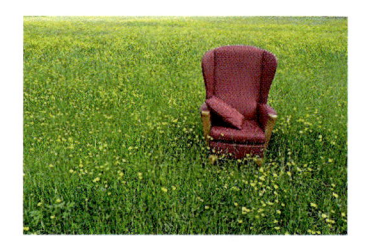

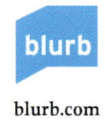

blurb.com

Me, my space, my place

Some personal experiences of a group of retired people who have made the move from 'home to Home'.

Compiled by
Maris Cole

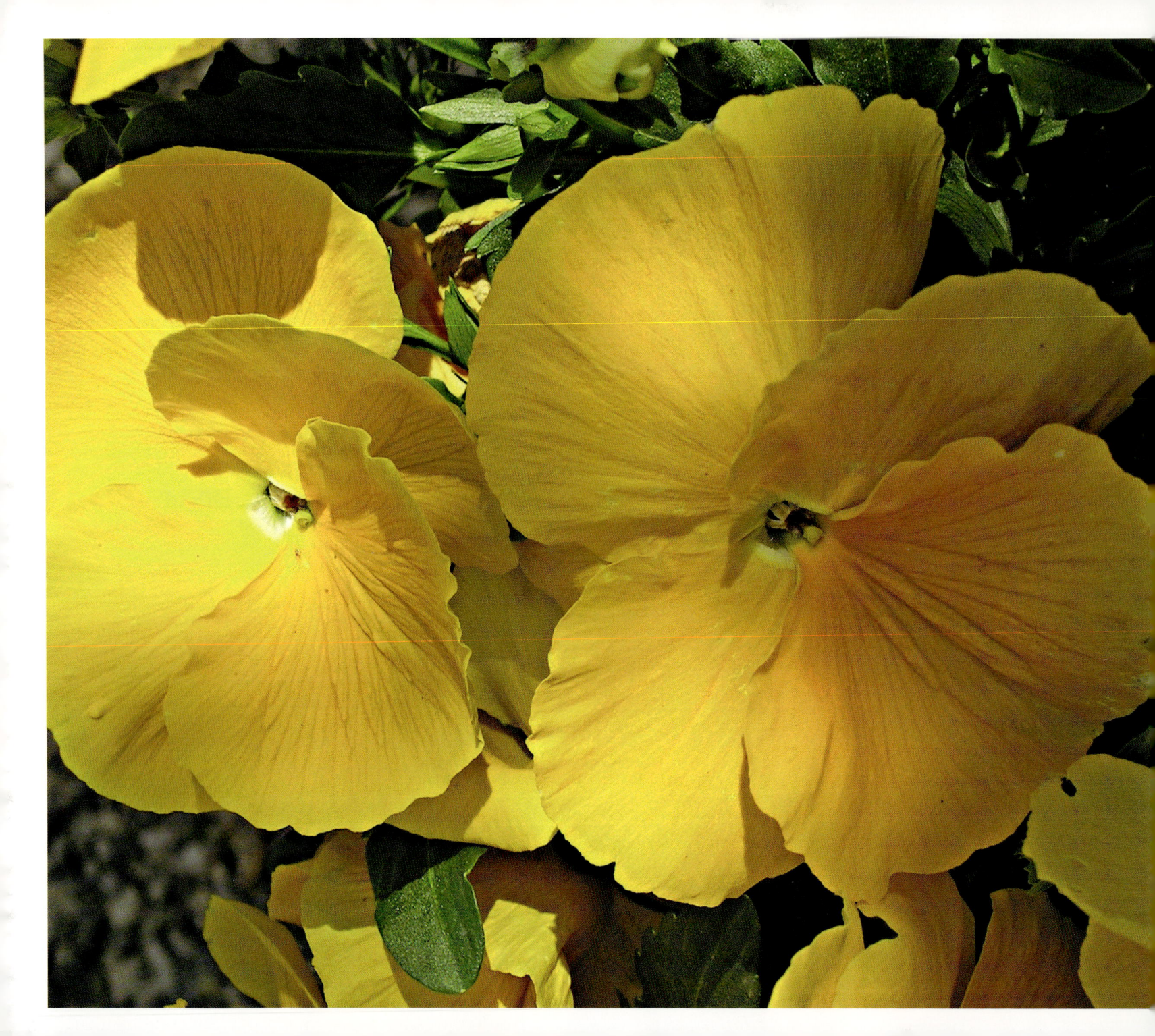

To move from one's own home into a residential Care Home is a major decision in life for many people.

This book is a collection of individual experiences, feelings and memories that were gathered during my quest to discover how people who retired to a Care Home in Malmesbury, Wiltshire made 'the Home *their* home'.

The people who so willingly shared their thoughts and opinions were some of the last residents to live in Burnham House before it closed and they moved into the new, purpose built Care Home, Athelstan House.

My journey of discovery with the residents revealed the individuality of each person and some of the influences on their lives at present and in the past. Our discoveries were realised through talking, listening, and sharing laughter and sorrows; often prompted by photographs, souvenirs or art activities.

Although all of the residents need care and support most of them want to be as independent as possible and try to achieve it in different and, sometimes, small ways.

Some residents personalise their room to create a microcosm of their own home and most have a collection of their own treasures and mementos that recall an earlier life. While some residents cherish their privacy; others do not want to be alone. Some people follow life-long interests and others look for new pleasures to enjoy.

All of these differences were accommodated and respected in Burnham House.

Several of the anecdotes about the past are reminders that these are the memories of a diminishing generation of people who started their young adult life during the second World War. Many of them served their country in the Armed Forces, in factories or on the land.

The combination of different life experiences, inner resources and personal day to day strategies revealed the individual ways that residents sustained themselves and made their lives and their place in Burnham House their own.

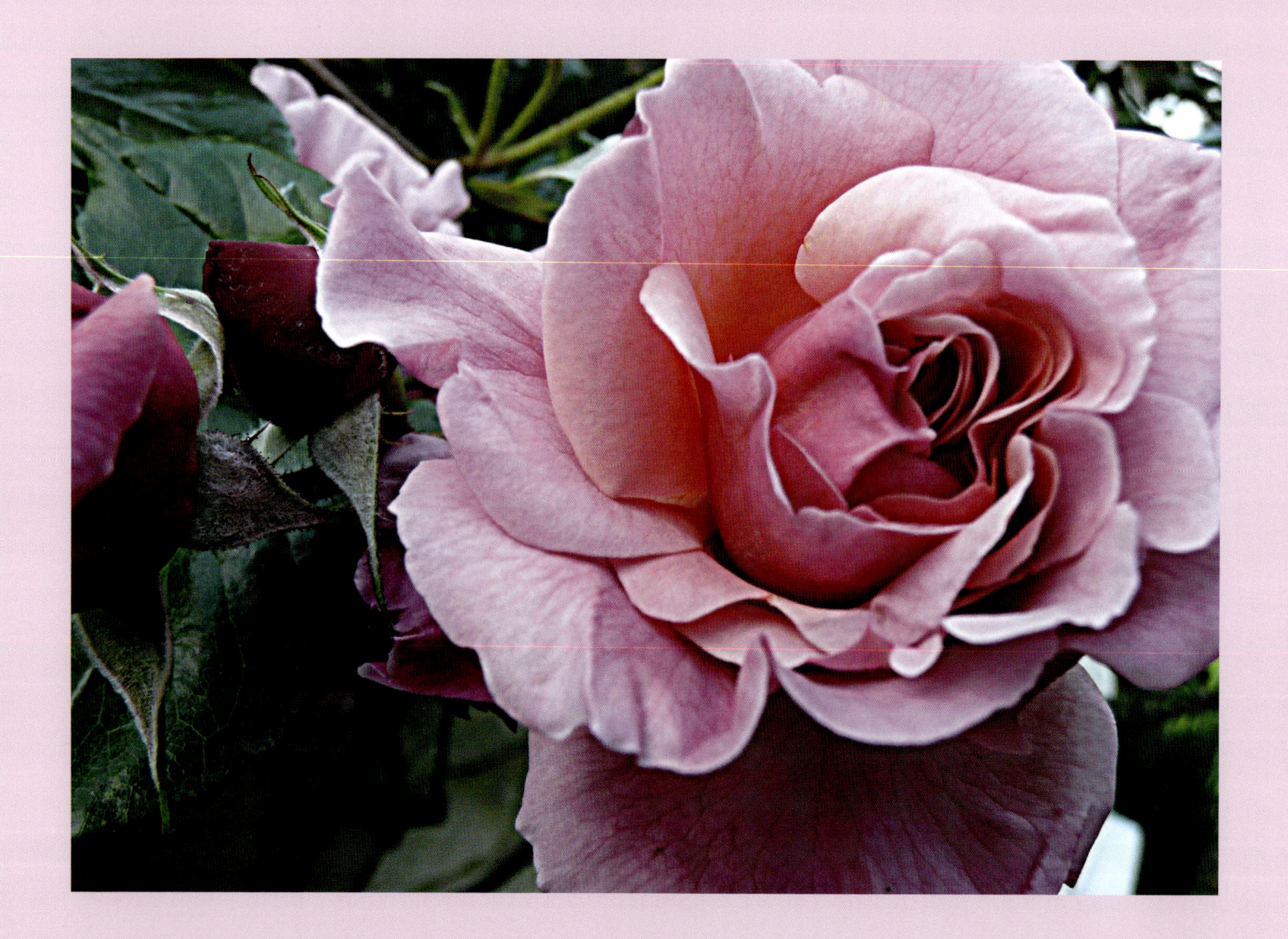

*'I wasn't ready
to be old.'*

Peggy

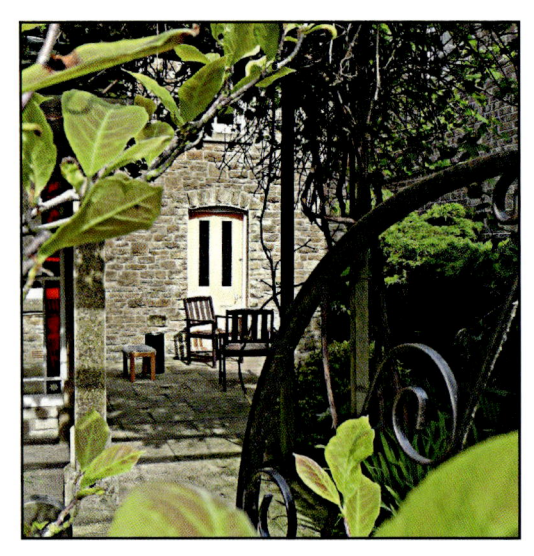

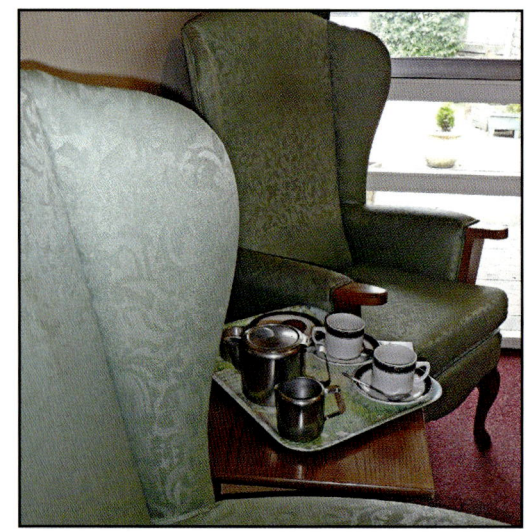

Peggy, why did you come to live here?
'When my husband died suddenly, it was a great shock and I don't think I have ever got over it. It was no good, I didn't like being on my own. I had a lot of brass and silver things that I used to clean. I decided I didn't want to do it anymore. I came to the Day Centre for one day a week, then two days, now I am living here. It's very friendly here and homely. **I like all the little corners and things about the place. It's cosy and snug.'**

How did you make your space your own place?

'It has helped having my own bed and furniture as well as my pictures, photographs and books.

My telephone is a real extravagance! *I've got a lot of very good friends and we like to keep in touch, some come to see me in the daytime.*

I'm not bored. I write letters, read magazines and I enjoy talking to people.'

Peggy takes part in many of the entertainments and activities at Burnham House and other places.

'I like the quizzes and have enjoyed sowing seeds and icing the Christmas cake. Some of us have been taken out for a drive and took flasks and some cake for a picnic.'

Roses on Peggy's pretty hand painted furniture

'I like music of all kinds and enjoy musicians and people coming to sing to us.
I love ballet. I used to dance when I was young, until I was about eighteen*. I like to go to the ballet at the Theatre Royal with my daughter. When my daughter was a child I used to keep the programmes and wrote on them when I took her to the ballet.*

I was a shorthand typist. I worked for all sorts of people and loved it. Shorthand was difficult to learn. I find I still do it when I am speaking on the telephone. I look down and see that I have written something in shorthand!'

Peggy Simpson

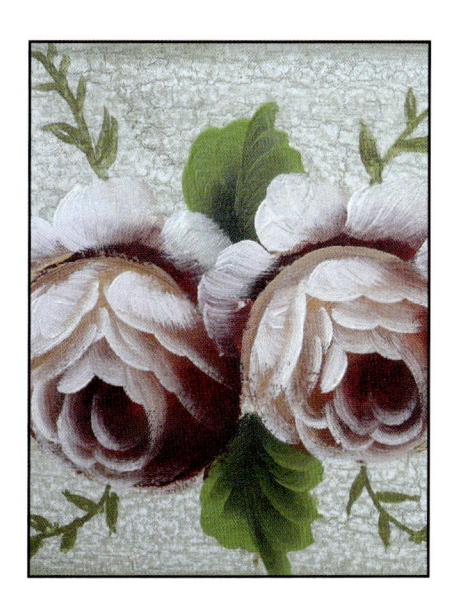

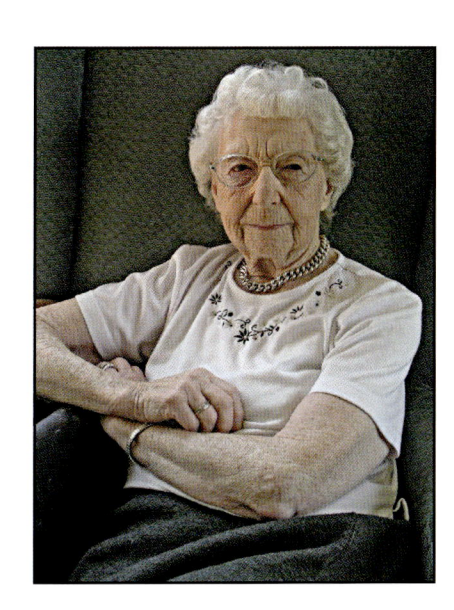

How have you made this place your home?

'I've always enjoyed my own company, that's the answer. I like to listen to the radio. I hate listening to music, I would rather listen to a talking book, a human voice. Talking books are delivered to me by the mobile library every month. I never get lonely. You don't think about that, being lonely, you think: well, what can I do next? In the afternoon I like to sit outside if it is fine and enjoy a cigarette. I love all the people here. I'm known and I get on with everybody. It's wonderful being here.

I used to be a professional magician. It was everything to me, to do a trick the way I liked to perform it. I had the gift of the gab, all the chat to go with the performance. I used to practise a trick over and over again for weeks to get it right. **I could pour a pint of milk into a handbag but I never pulled a rabbit out of a hat!'**

In his mid-thirties John was a badly injured victim in a car accident.
'My life stopped. *But I consider myself lucky, it could have been worse.'*

John Parsons

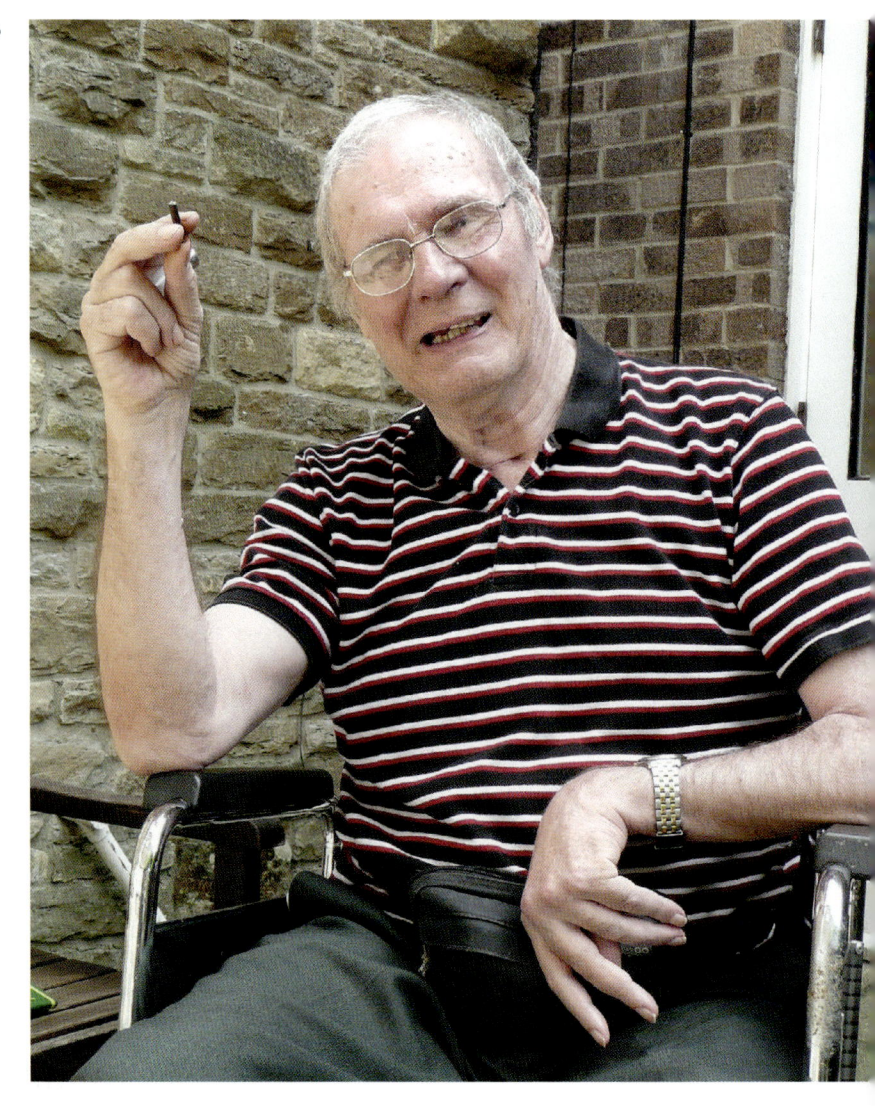

Reita and a friendly visitor.

Reita enjoys being in company so likes to spend time in the lounge.

When her husband, Bruce, was breeding race horses Reita used to help with the young foals. She is very good with animals.

Reita was a very active person and still enjoys the opportunity to dance when there is a party.

She rode regularly and was a keen gardener who especially liked growing flowers. As a farmer's wife she helped on their farm and when they were very busy, or when staff were ill, Reita helped with the milking.

Reita Akerman

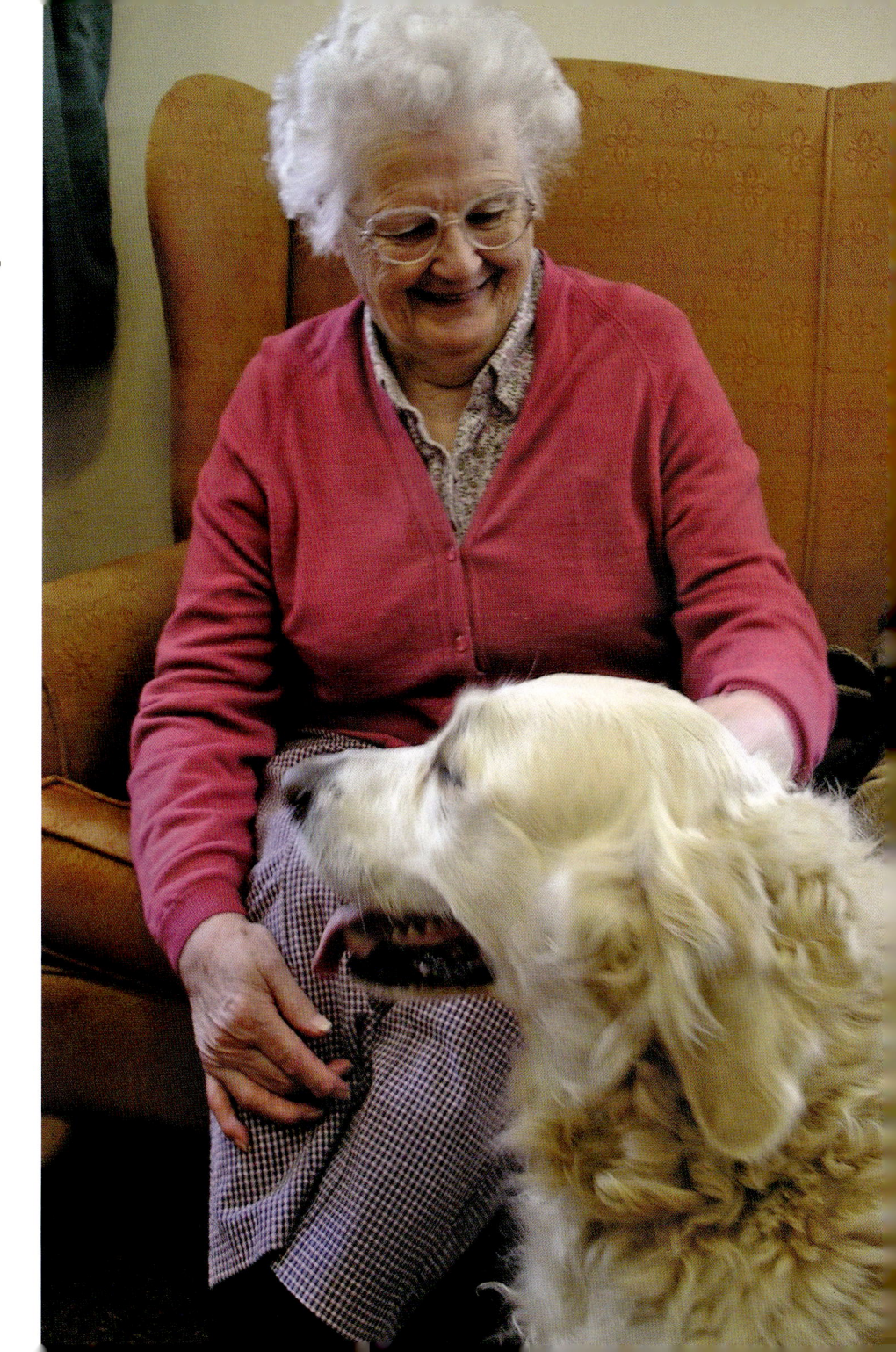

Geoffrey keeps a kindly eye on everyone.

'It is nice here. Burnham House is a homely place.'

Do you have a favourite place here?

'I like to sit in the lounge because I can see what is going on. I don't stay in my room because I like being with people.

Also if I am in the lounge I can get to the dining room easily on my own.

It is nice to see someone. My sister and my sister-in-law come to visit me every week. They bring me cake or some fruit. My sister-in-law looked after me after I had a stroke before I came to live here.'

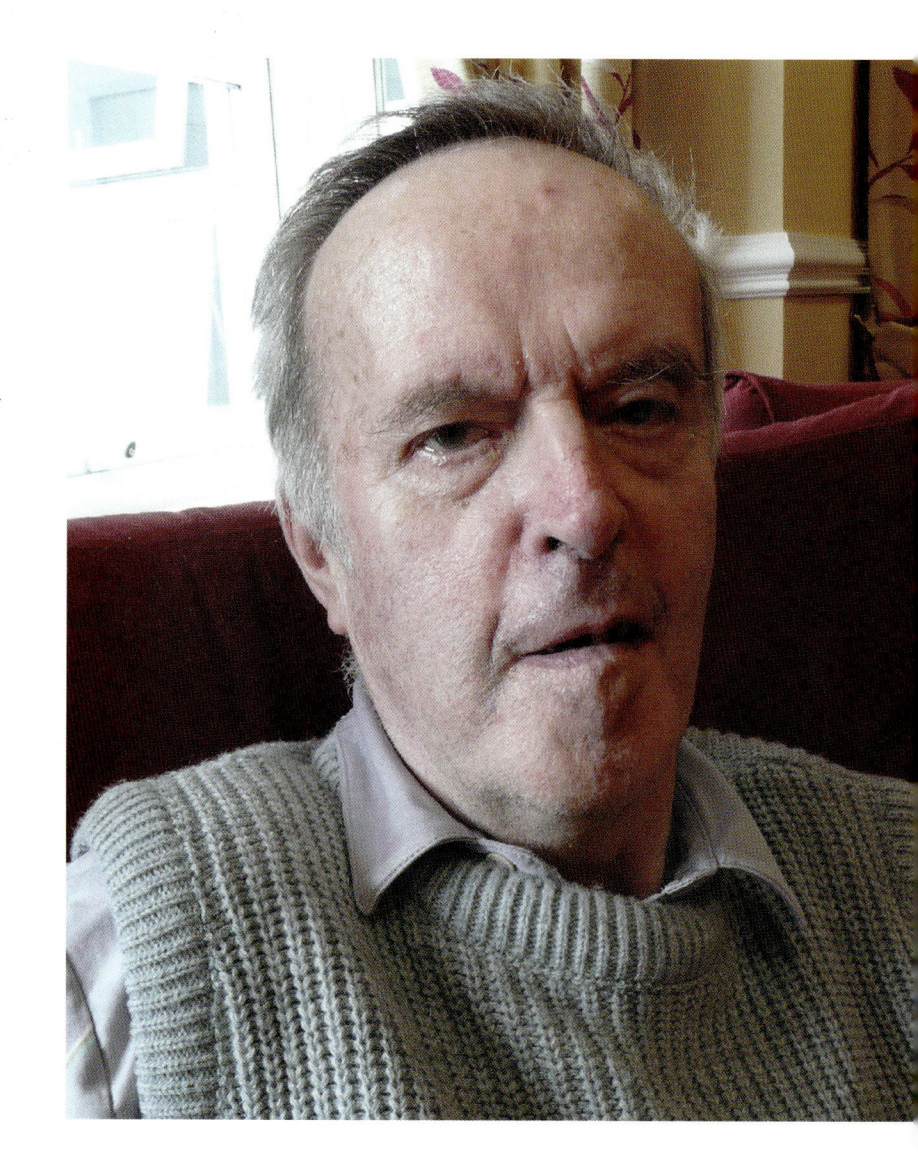

'In my room I have some pictures of racehorses and a statue of a horse. I didn't ride myself but I worked for Lord Oaksey who was a racing commentator. **The Oaksey family gave me this picture when I retired.**'

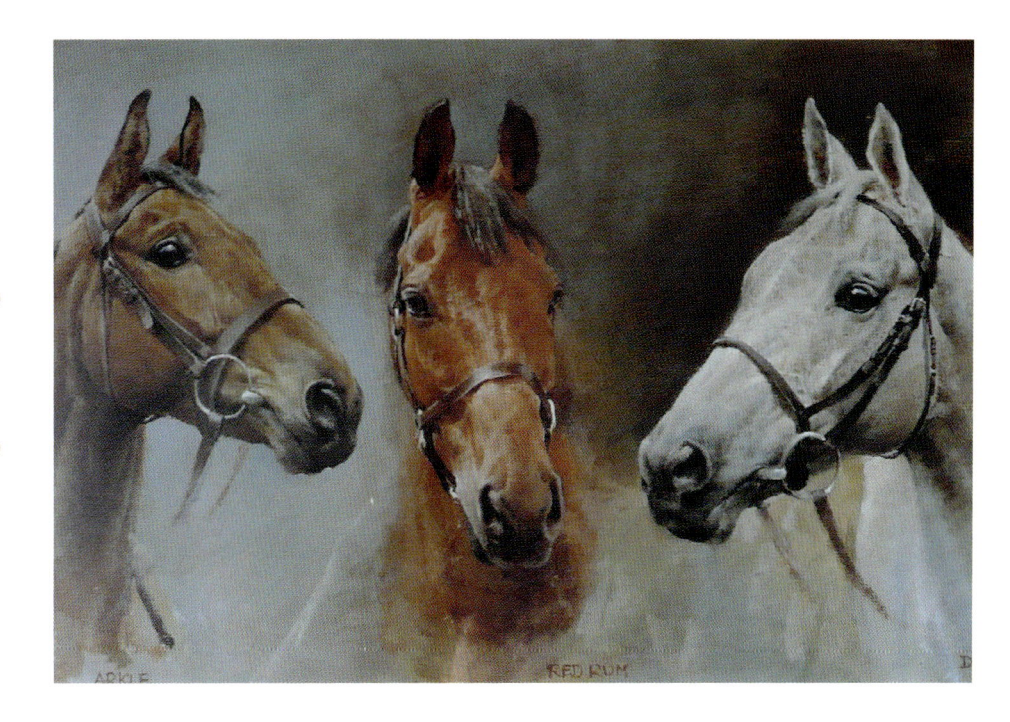

Arkle, Red Rum and Desert Orchid

What did you do when you worked?

*'I worked for Lord Oaksey at Hill Farm in Oaksey for fifty two years. I was the handyman outdoors. I cycled to work and my first job was to collect the daily papers from the village shop.
Next I took the dogs, four Jack Russells, for a walk. I liked doing this best and walked for about two miles.*

If they needed a fire in the house I would get the logs in.

We had a little room where I cleaned the shoes brought down for me then I left them in the passage. Usually I had a cup of coffee in the kitchen with the person who did the housework. Lady Oaksey often joined us.

We had a gardener so I collected the vegetables that he grew and sometimes helped prepare them for the cook. I did the lawnmowing and walked with the very big mower. Round at the stables my job was to take the muck away.'

Geoffrey Boulton

'I have made my room my home'

Dorothy

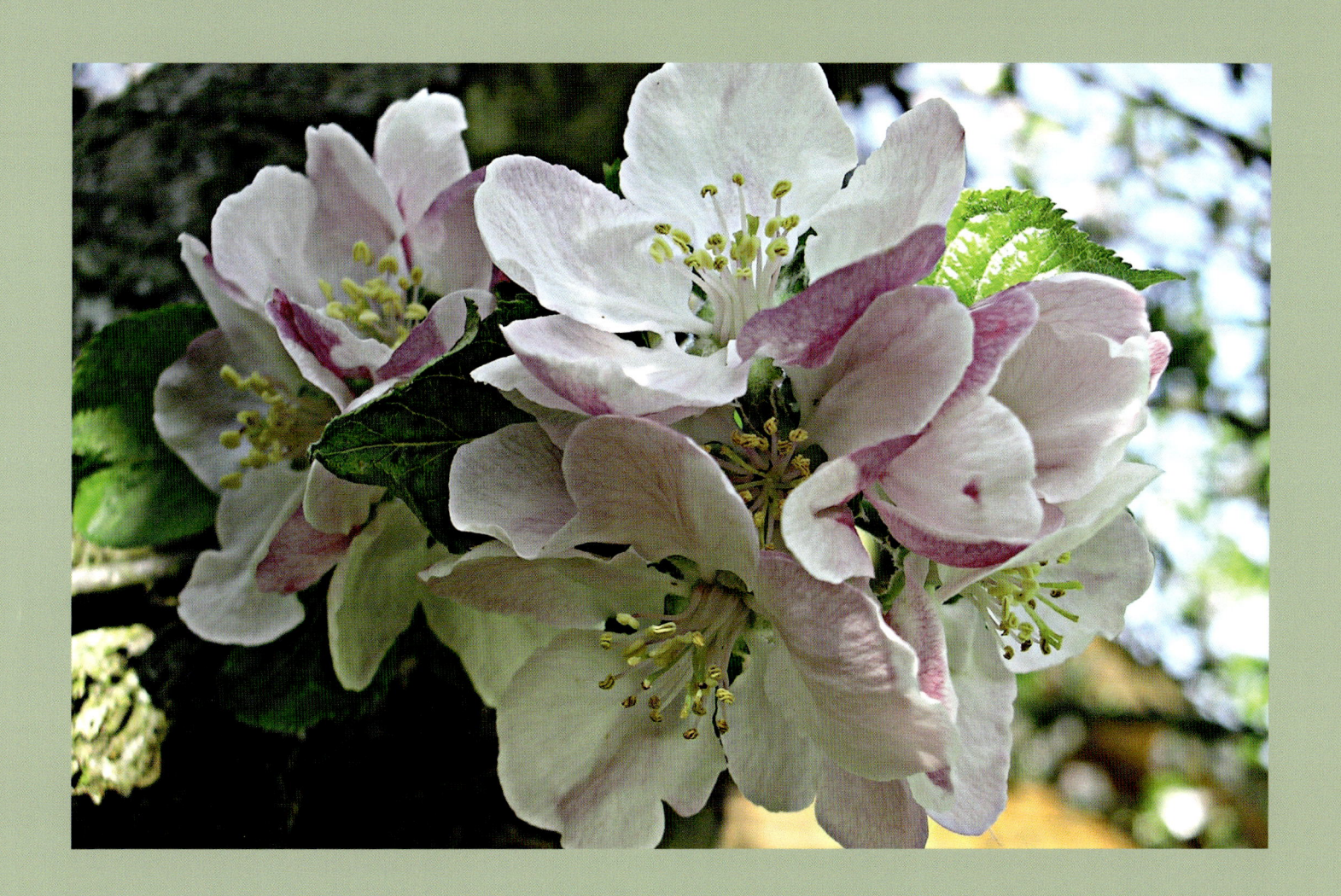

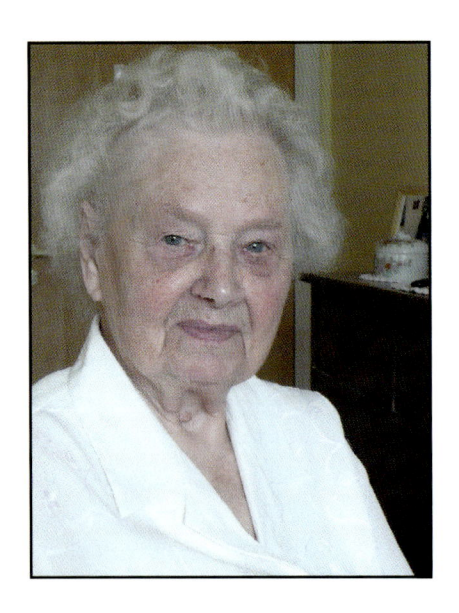

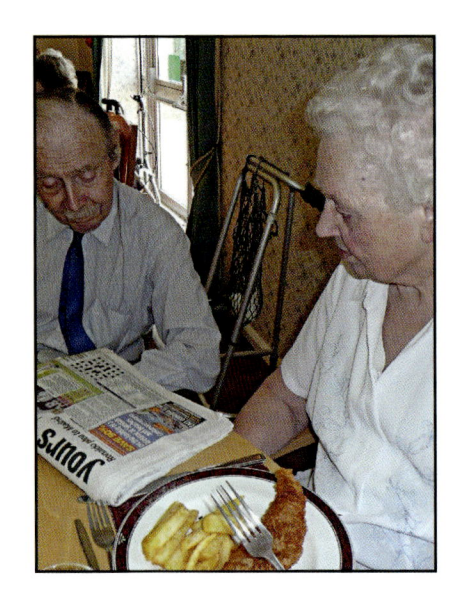

Peggy came to live at Burnham House in 1991

'I brought some of my own furniture from home for my room. **I have a chest of drawers made by my grandfather who was a carpenter by trade.** Also I have a sewing box and my own china cabinet for photographs and ornaments.

I am quite happy in my own company and don't need entertaining all the time.

I would be lost without a book. You can pick it up and put it down whenever you like. I have a daily paper and do the crossword puzzles. We compare notes at lunchtime asking:

"What did you get for this or that?"

I have breakfast in my room but go to the dining room for my lunch and tea.
In my room I enjoy listening to the radio and find it soothing to knit and listen to the radio at the same time.

It is nice to see people. All my children live in Malmesbury so I see them at weekends. I go to lunch with my sons and I see my grandchildren.

I have been on some of the outings organised by the staff and I enjoyed going to the Luncheon Club held in the Town Hall. Also I enjoy going to the Handicap Club in Malmesbury. It is a social get together where we have quizzes and do exercises and occasionally go to a garden for afternoon tea.'

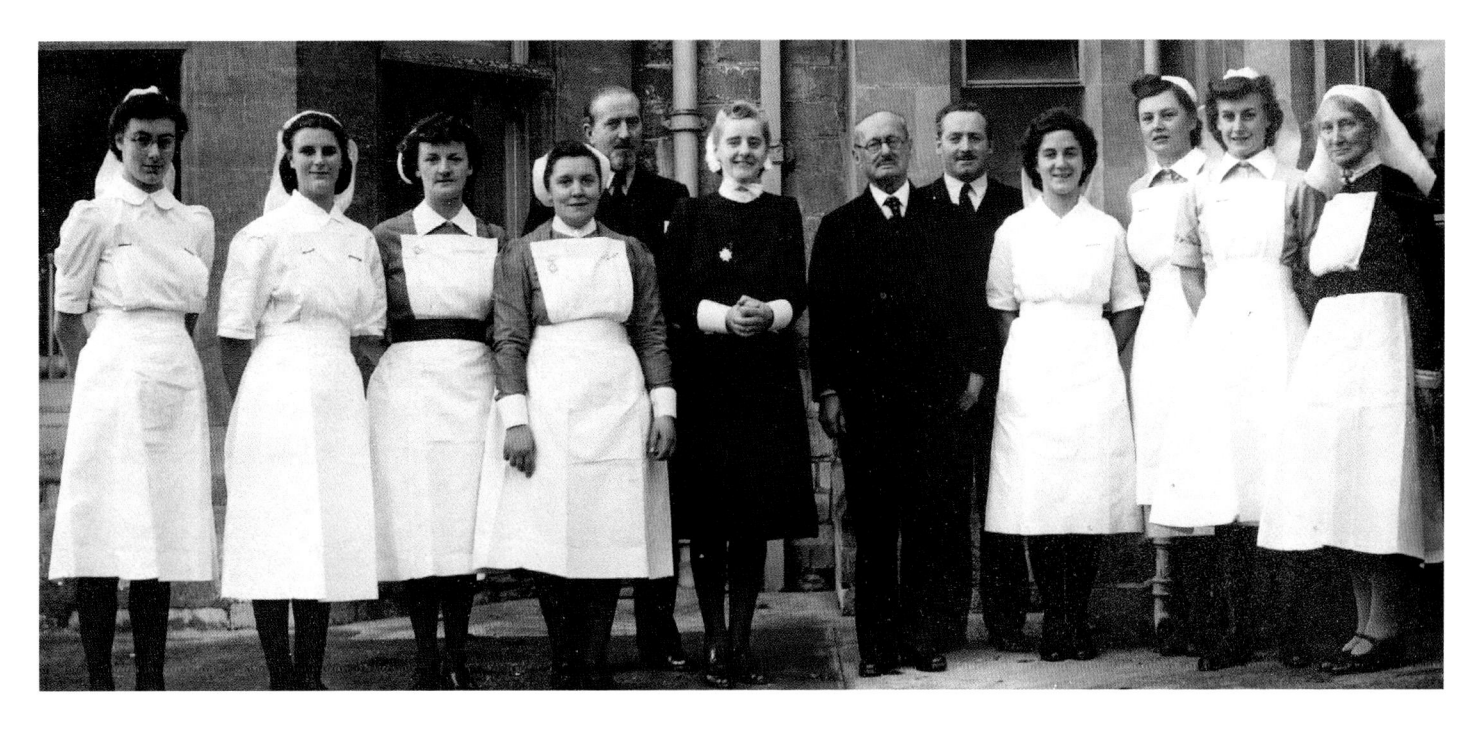

Peggy, third from the right, at the opening of the first extension to Malmesbury Hospital by Lord Horder

Peggy worked as nurse for over thirty years before she retired from Westhill Nursing Home in Malmesbury.
'In 1945 I came from Bristol to work at Tetbury Maternity Hospital on Gumstool Hill. Mark Phillips was born there. It was hard work and golly, our feet hurt going up and down those stone stairs!

Three days after the babies were born they were looked after in the nursery downstairs. Our uniforms and accommodation were paid for and our rooms were up in the original attics. I worked there for five years then moved to Malmesbury Hospital because it was a training hospital until the National Health Service started in 1948.
We had some fun at Christmas in Malmesbury Hospital. The roast turkey was brought into the front hall and the doctor used to carve it. We dashed around with the food, taking the Christmas dinner to the patients.'

Peggy Pike

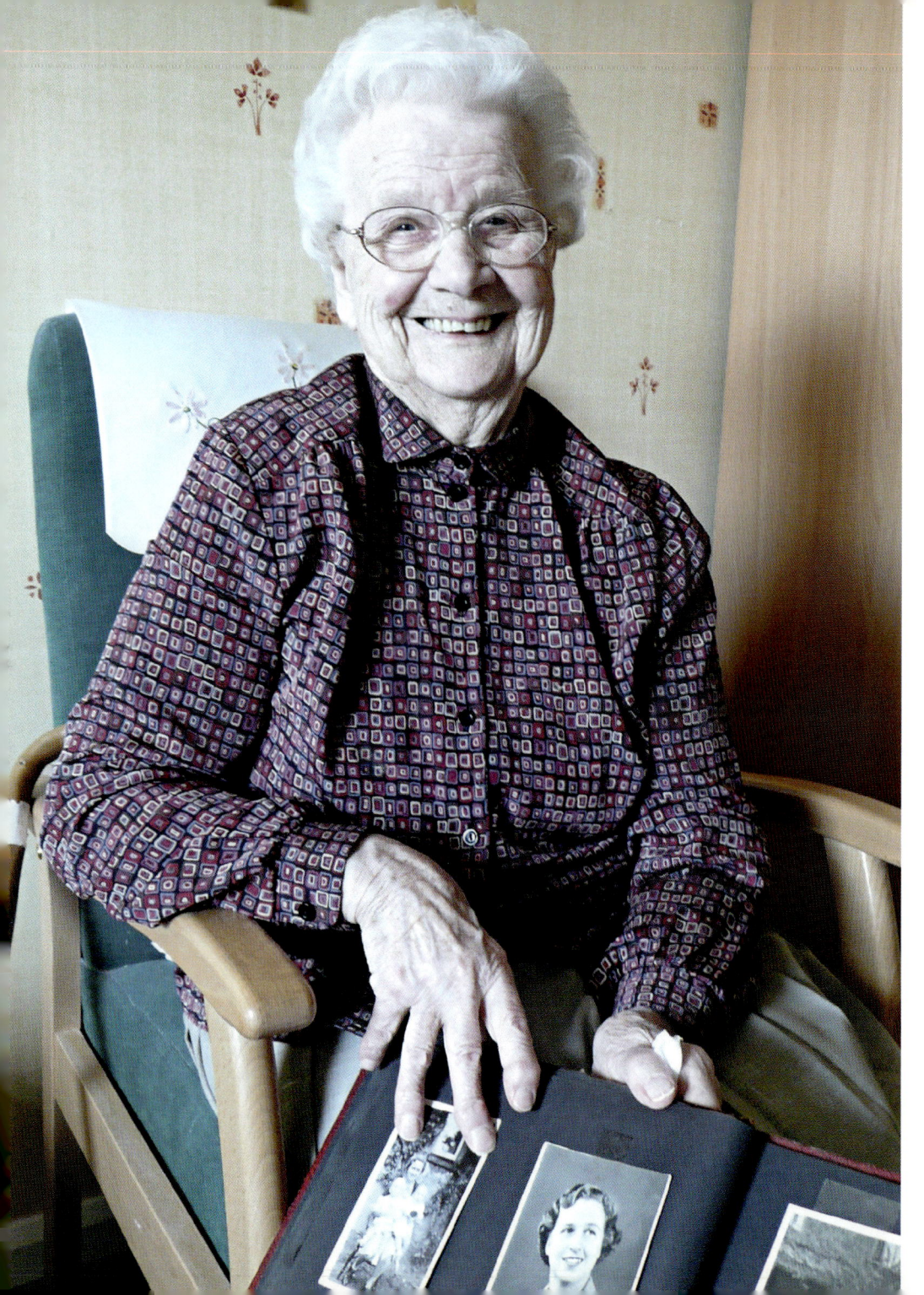

'I am quite content and happy on my own,' says Dorothy.

'I am a "loner" in a way but I'm never miserable. In the morning I sit back and relax in my room.
I don't like a lot of people around me but I leave my door open to see people passing by. I'm not nosey but I like to know people are there. I can't bear to be shut in.
I sometimes go to the lounge in the afternoon until about half past three, then I go to my room to watch television before tea. I'm not one for going out a lot but I've been on several trips. Occasionally I have been taken out for a drive to a coffee morning.
I have enjoyed going out with someone I can have a conversation with.'

'I take great care of all of my things. I am very proud of them especially the tapestry cushions I made myself.'

Did you work when you were younger?

'In my younger years I was a real nanny. In those days you weren't accepted as a nanny unless you had trained under a head nanny. **I first started as a nursery maid with a uniform and cap and everything.** I did that for two years. The head nanny wore a white pique frock and sat in a chair giving her orders. I had to carry all the meals up from the kitchen to the nursery.

There were four children and every year we went with them for a month's holiday. We went to the Lake District and Bognor Regis and stayed in a rented house. The parents didn't come with us, they only had the children with them between one and two o'clock every day at home but not on holiday.'

Dorothy Pooley

Dorothy and her charges, Catherine and David, on holiday in Porthcawl.

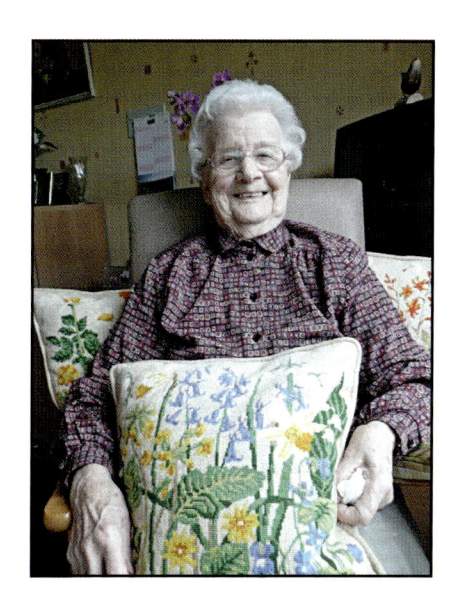

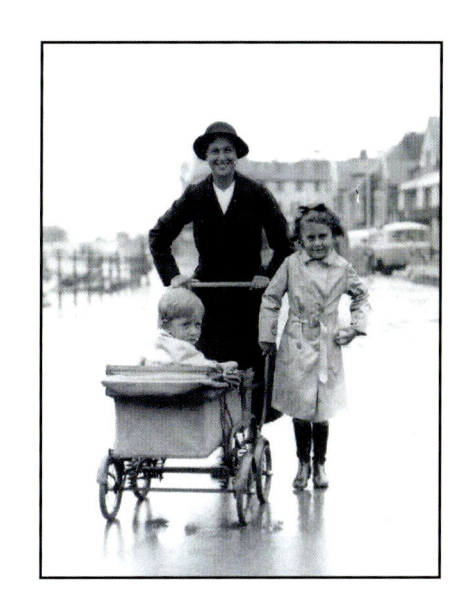

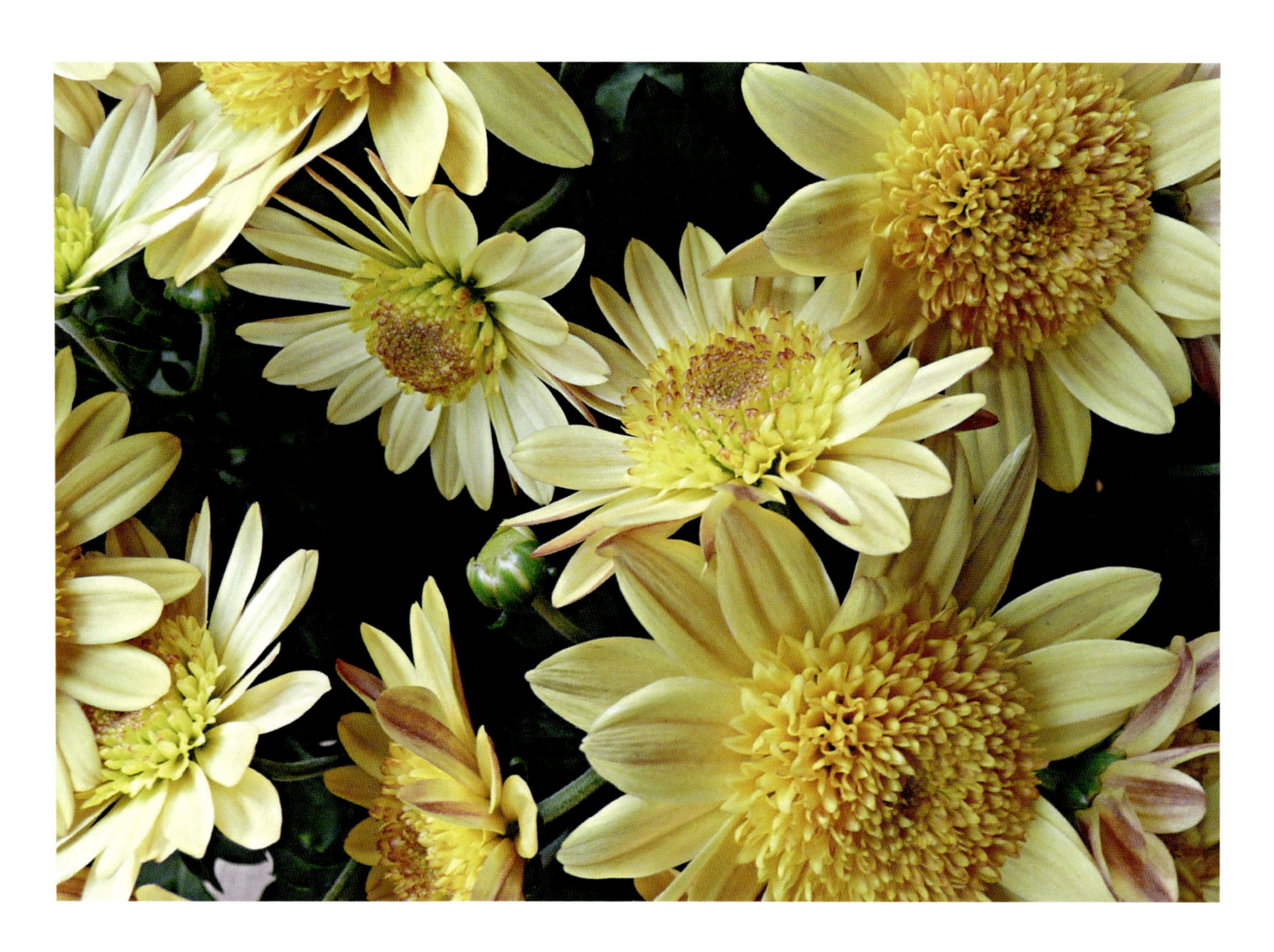

'I could be content here.'

Marjorie

Sidney has been interested in sport all of his life.

'I like to spend some time in my room because I enjoy watching sport on television.

If I was on my own at home I know that I couldn't cope.
*If I hadn't come here to live I would have found it very difficult to ask my family for help if I needed it. My son lives in Essex and my daughter lives in New Zealand so we cannot see each other very often.
I would be such a terrible nuisance to them and **I like to be independent.***
I am very lucky because I have had a good life although I had a spell of bad health.

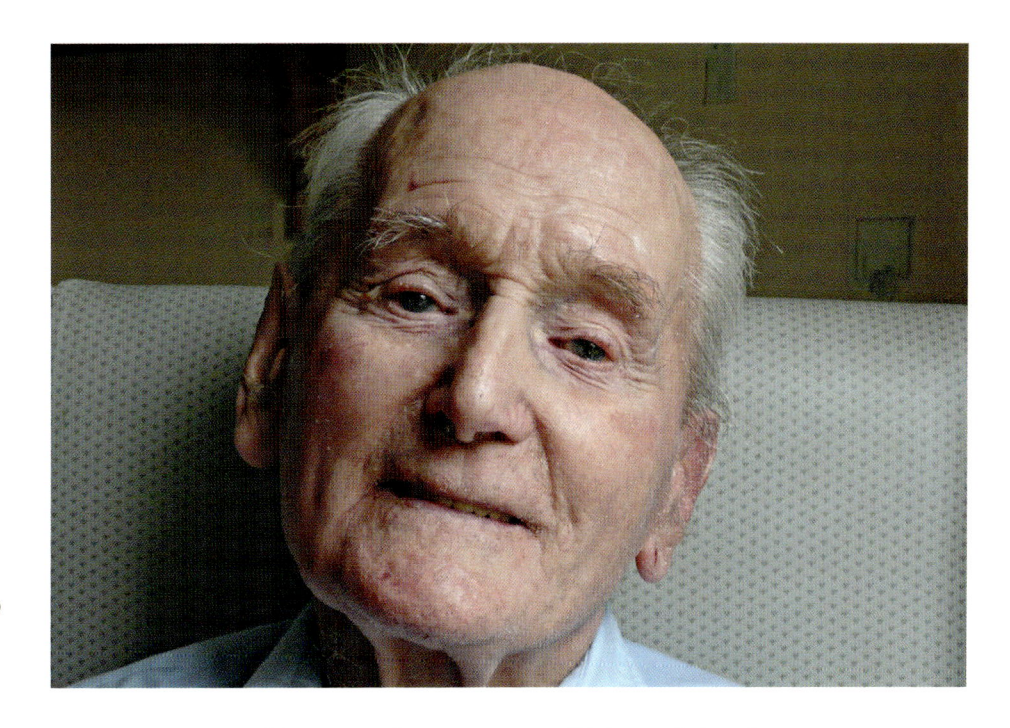

Ex-marathon runner Sidney Lloyd

I was born in 1915. I loved sport especially running. For a number of years I used to do a baker's round. I pulled the barrow by hand and it was hard work. After work I used to run in Richmond Park. The keeper let me keep my bicycle near his house. I ran twice around the park and that was fifteen miles altogether. I never got fed up with it. Running was a sporting challenge for me. I entered some marathons and as well as running I played football and was a keen tennis player. It all came naturally to me.
If I could go back to the age of twenty five it would be wonderful!'

Freddie chose the things he wanted to keep with him when he moved from Dorset to Burnham House.

'My son arranged the pictures in my room. **Photographs and pictures are easily moved. They have been taken from place to place during my life and quickly help to make a place familiar, more like home.** I used to be a keen photographer, mainly landscapes and buildings. I had a darkroom for developing my prints and found that to be the most interesting part of the process.

This oil painting was painted by my wife Kathleen.'

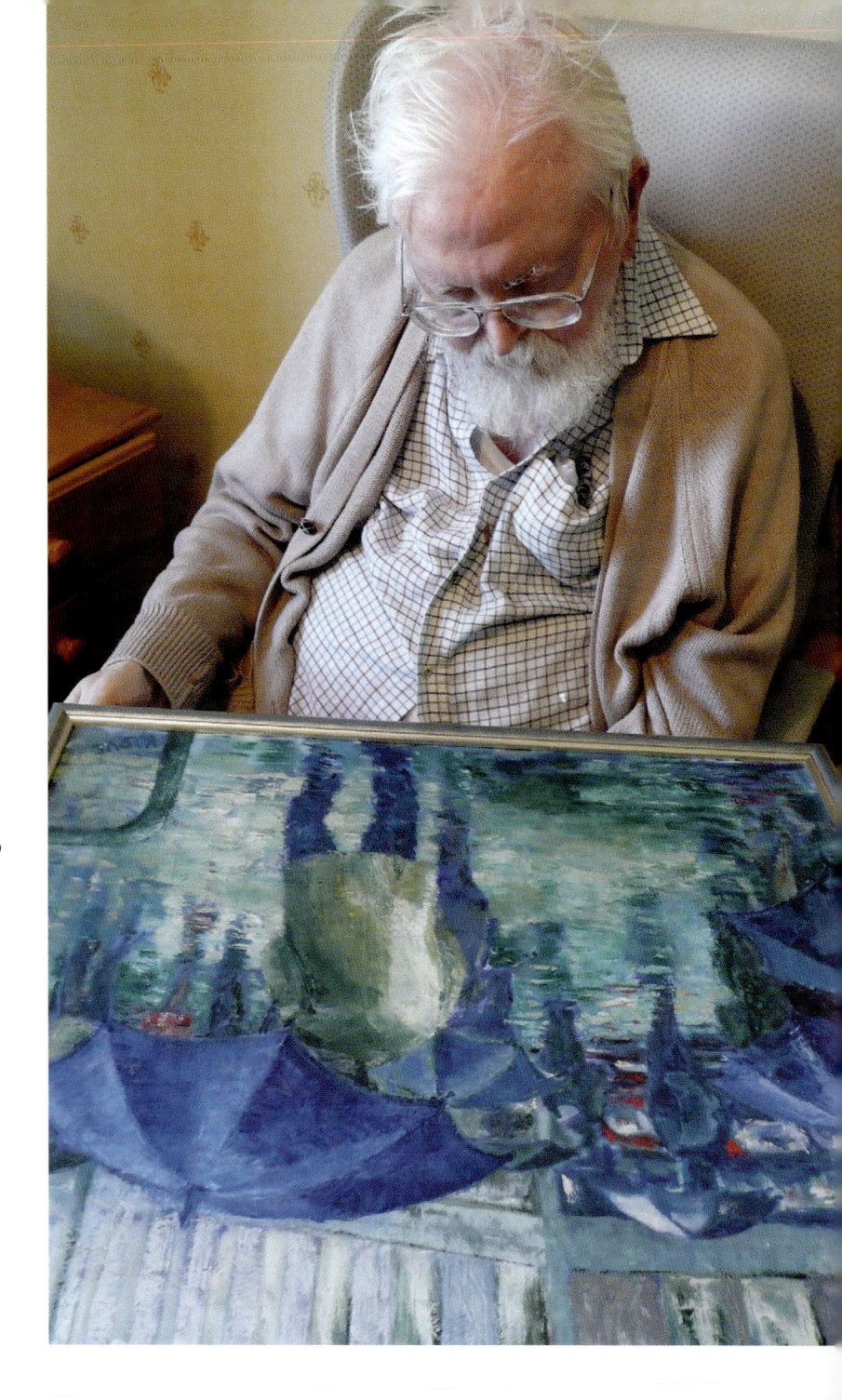

'Radio 4 is my standby.'

'I am in my room most of the day. It would be nice to have people you could have a conversation with but Radio 4 is my standby.
I enjoy historical and scientific programmes.
I cannot read easily so visitors are important to me. **Something I really like is the Talking Books from the Blind Association.** The service is excellent. They send me a list and I choose one at a time.
I make quite a lot of use of the telephone. I speak to my family and one or two friends from the past. I would really like to be able to use a computer and e-mail facility.
I have been on some outings while I have been here. When I went to the Gloucester Waterways Museum I enjoyed a pleasant afternoon on a canal boat and we took a picnic. When that kind of outing is offered, that is when I go.'

Freddie Love is experienced at making a home in new places.
'I joined the Foreign Diplomatic Service straight from Cambridge University. My first posting was bewildering. My wife and I had just got married in 1952 and I was posted to Istanbul. There was always a lot of business involved in finding somewhere to live that fitted the rent allowance. We were posted every four years. Working in the embassies was the most interesting, dealing with trade agreements, relations with foreign powers and cultural exchanges. Work in the consulate, that looks after British interests and citizens' visas, was less interesting.'

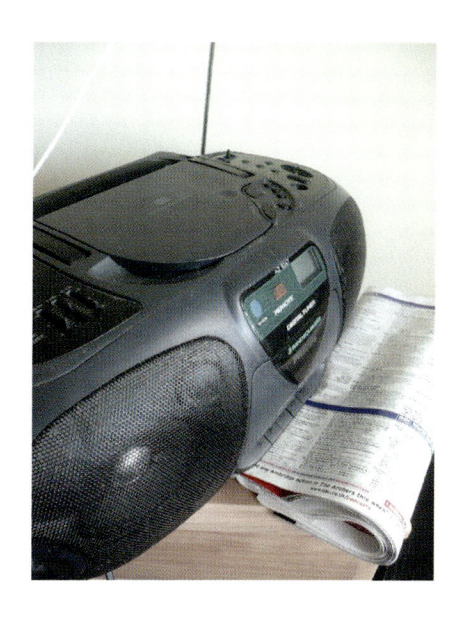

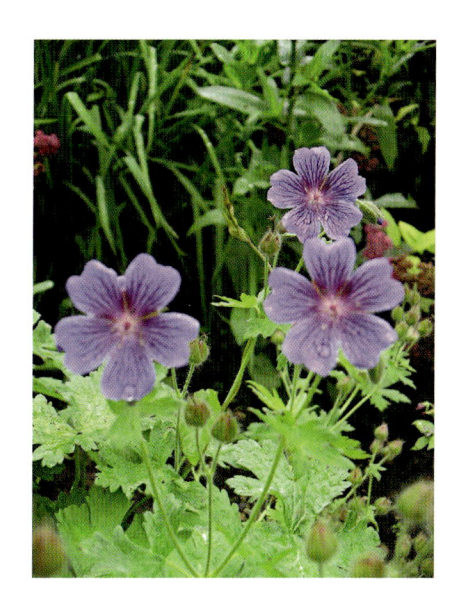

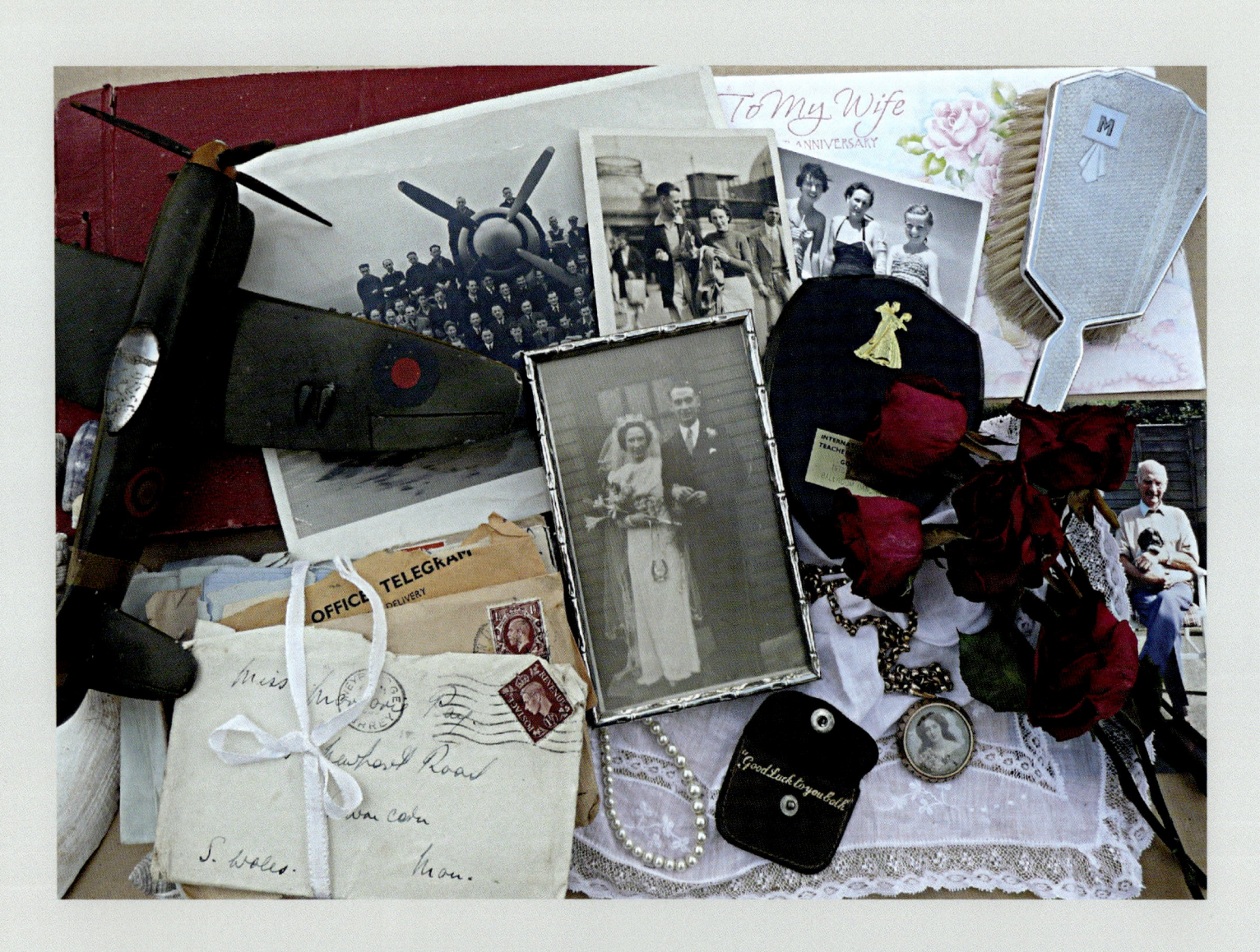

Treasures, remembrances and souvenirs...

'In my room I have some nice pieces of china. This little cat is sweet, the sauciest little thing. I bought it at a sale here.'

Lottie used to work as a shorthand typist and book keeper.

'When I first started work I cycled but I learned to drive when I was in my twenties. I had an Austin 12 car. My husband taught me to drive but we didn't fall out. He told me, "You do as I say, mind." So I did as I was told.'

As a child Lottie went to the village school in Burton. She remembers an Inspector's visit when he told this story:

The cuckoo comes in April
He sings a song in May

He gives us a tune
In the middle of June

In July he flies away
And in August
Go he must.

'I am happy here. The girls are cheerful, that makes a lot of difference. They are all very kind to me.

When I look out of my window it looks lovely in the Courtyard, it is so pretty. *When I had a place of my own I loved gardening. In your own place you always find something to do.
I don't go into the lounge very often. I enjoy being in my room where I sometimes listen to the wireless or read. I watch television most. I like "Flog It!", "Coronation Street" and "Emmerdale"; I tried watching "Eastenders" but it was so dreary.*

I have been on some of the trips. I enjoyed going to Lydiard Park because I hadn't been there before.'

Lottie Andrews

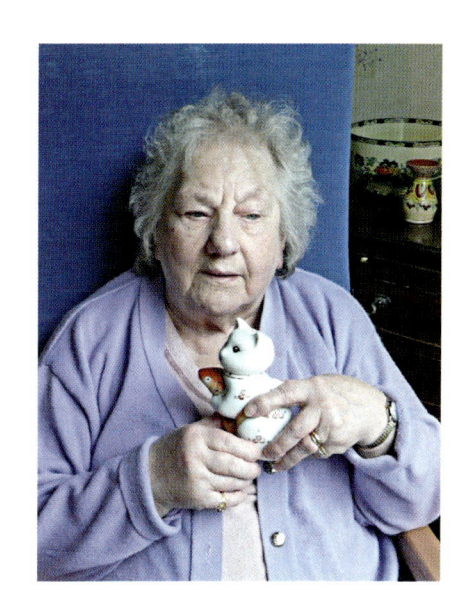

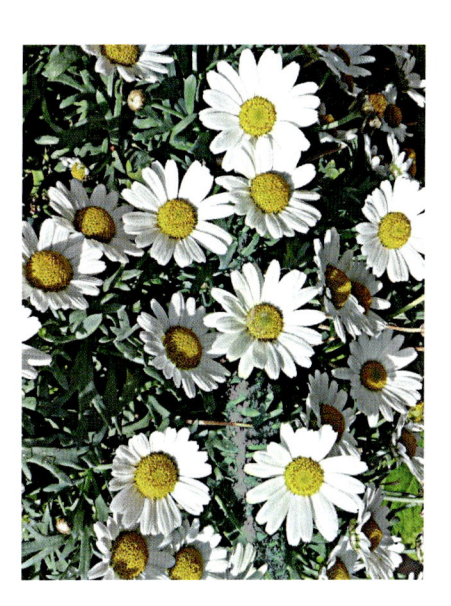

Listening to music is one of Greta's pleasures.

'I like the radio and listening to music on my own downstairs.

*Also I like to see gardens but I'm a bit wobbly on my legs. We used to have a lovely flower garden at home. My parents used to cut some flowers to take to church every Sunday. I liked doing **some** gardening. I would say to my father and brothers, "Would you like a weeder?" and they said, "Yes, you look like one."*

This tapestry picture shows the fountain in the Market Square in Wiener Neustadt where we used to do our shopping.'

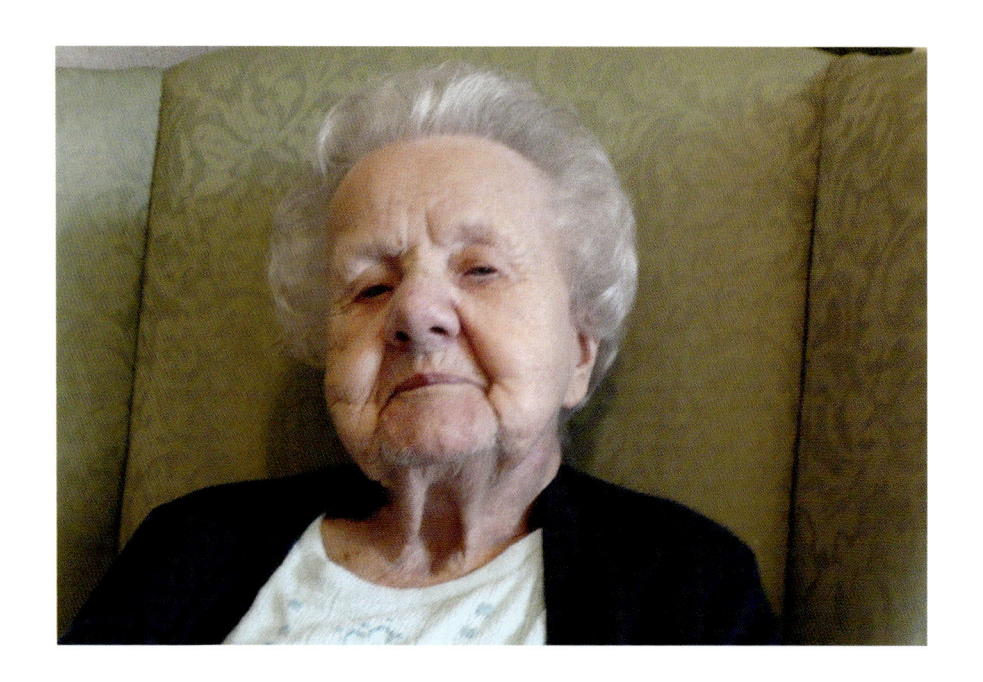

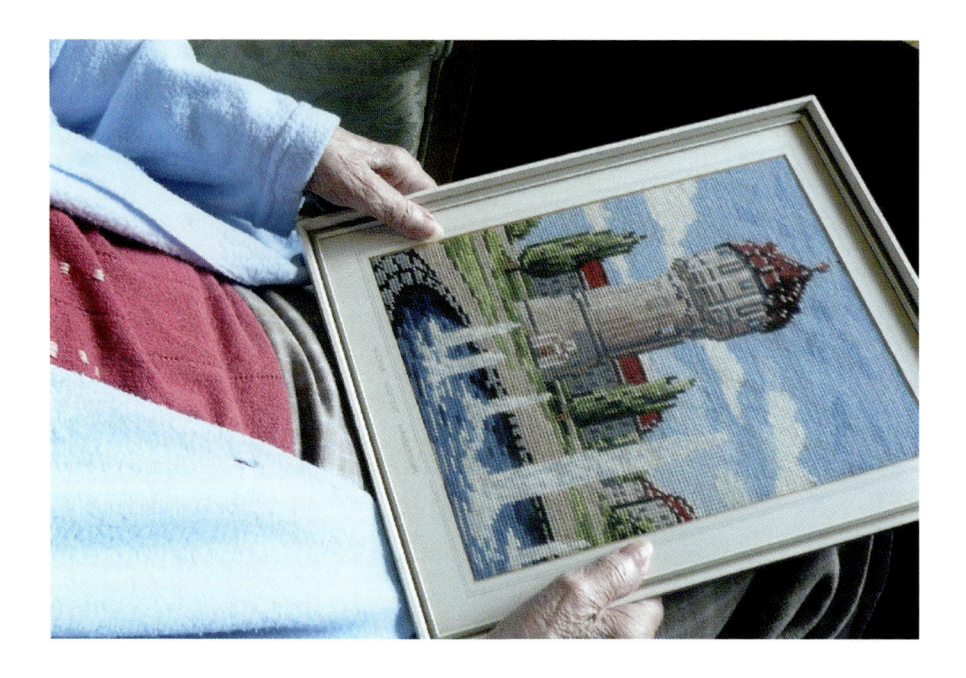

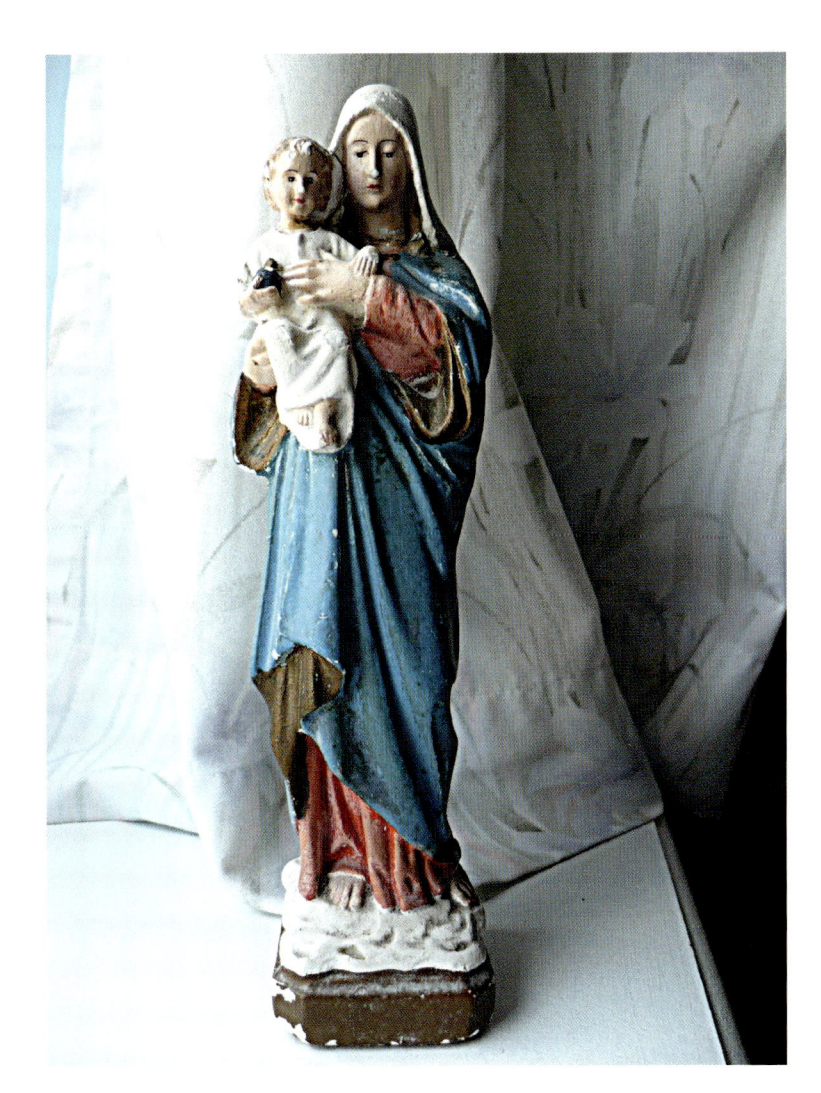

This Madonna is a lovely remembrance for Greta.

'My parents gave it to me to take for my room when I left home. My mother said,
"Take that with you because it will remind you of home." '

Greta grew up in the town of Wiener Neustadt, Austria, but came to England to work in domestic service.

*'I had a young man but he died.
I waited and waited; I got older and older and did more and more work.'*

Greta Verinda

Peggy used to be a secretary.
'I enjoyed working because I liked being with people. That's why I like being downstairs. I don't talk much but I like to see what is going on. **This is the Taj Mahal.** *It belonged to my grandfather but I don't know if he went there.'*
                                                      Peggy Murphy

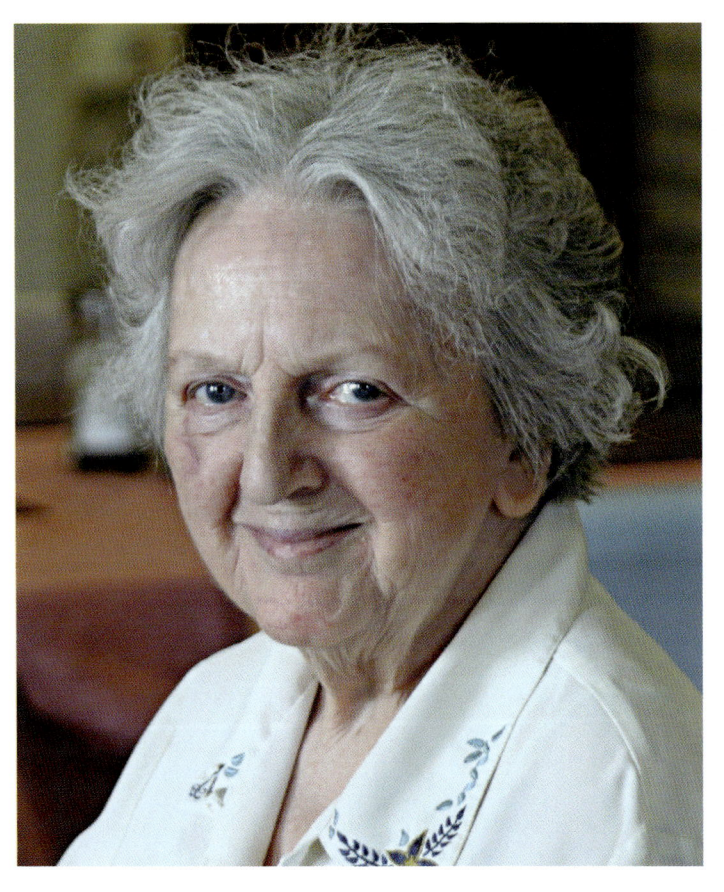

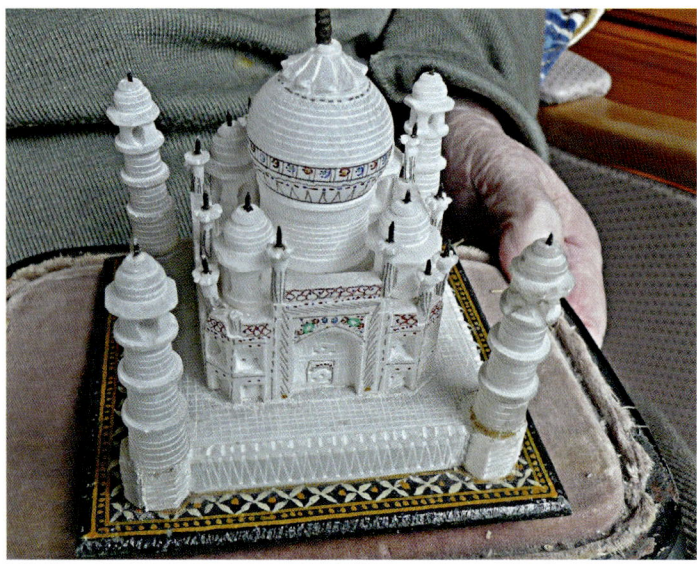

'I didn't have a teddy when I was young, I always wanted one and now I have one with me in my room.'

Queenie Riley

'This chair is important to me because it came from home and is part of my home here. I brought my mantel clock and my wireless because I like to listen to the wireless when I go to bed.

I have a newspaper every day. My eyesight is poor but I can read the large print. I like to go to the lounge where I sit and listen so that I know what is going on. **A sense of humour, that's something you mustn't lose.** Everything is done for you here but I like to do things for myself really. I like to go out especially to new places.

At home, knitting, sewing and gardening were my three loves.'

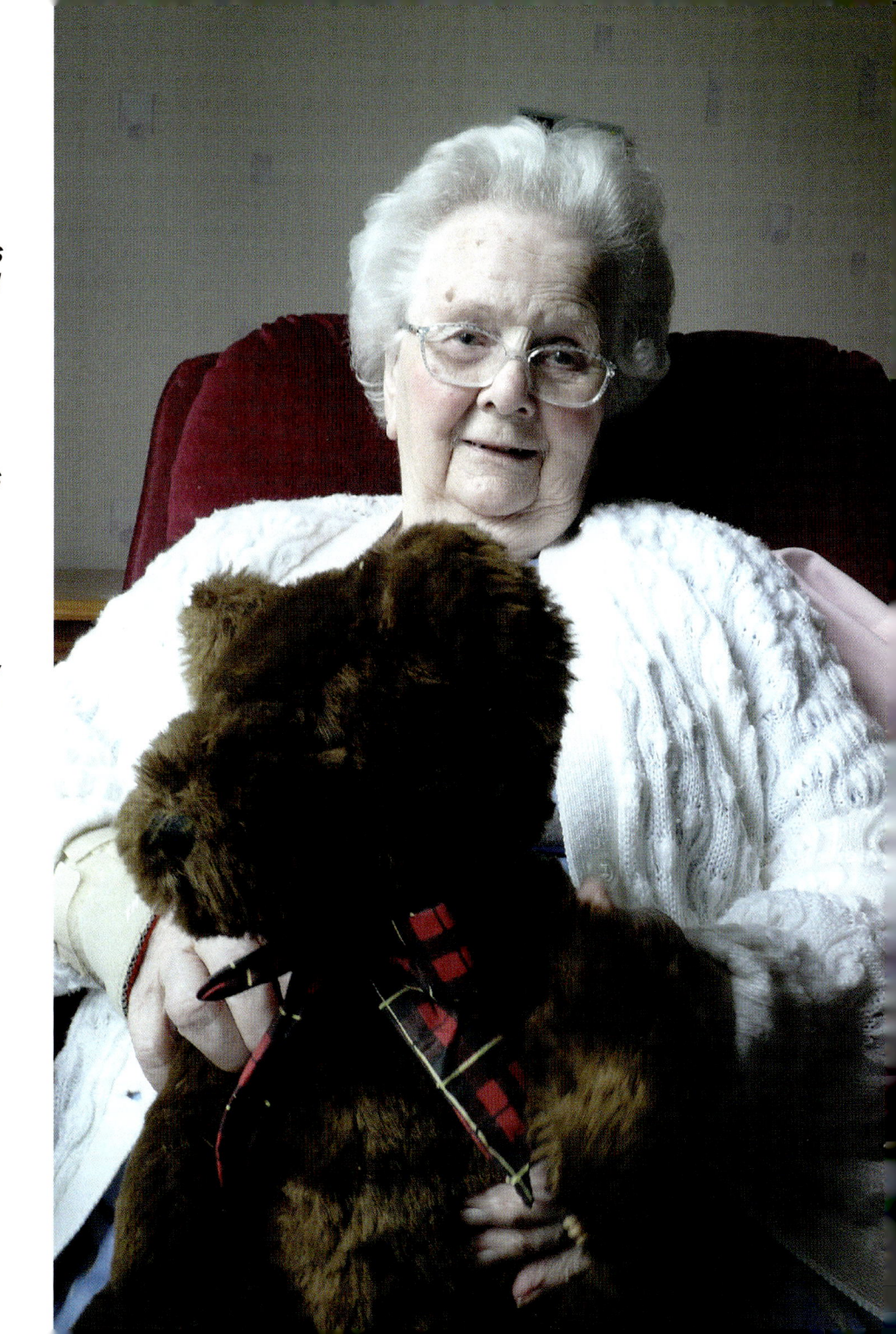

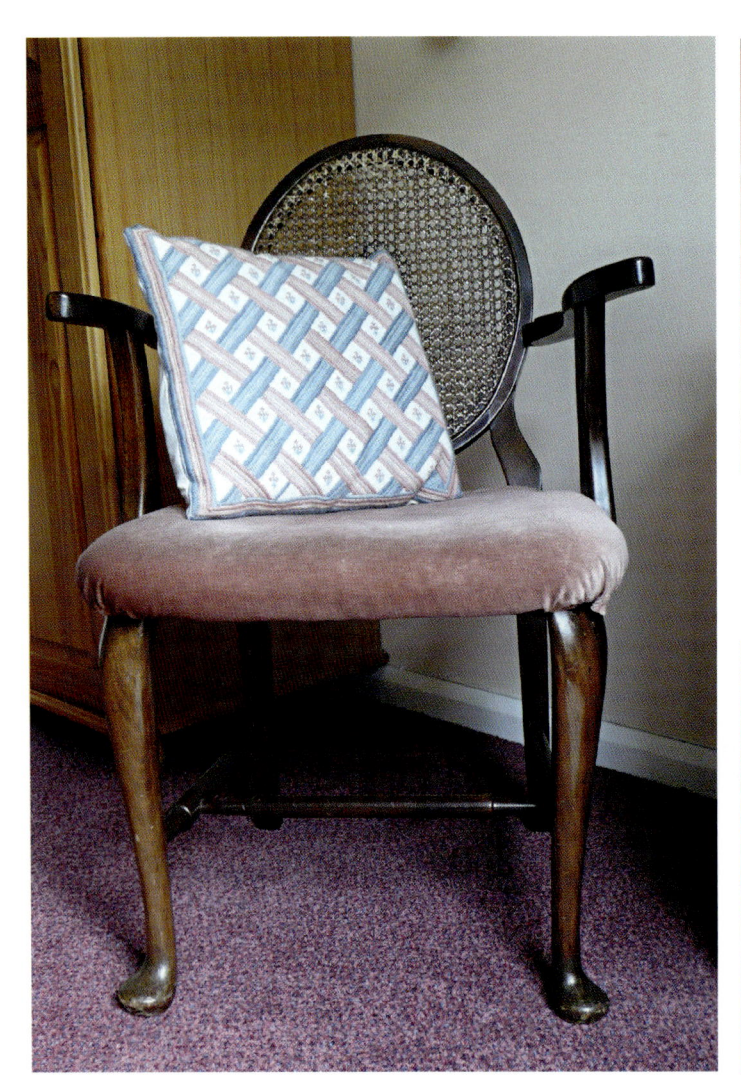

'I have some of my own things from home,

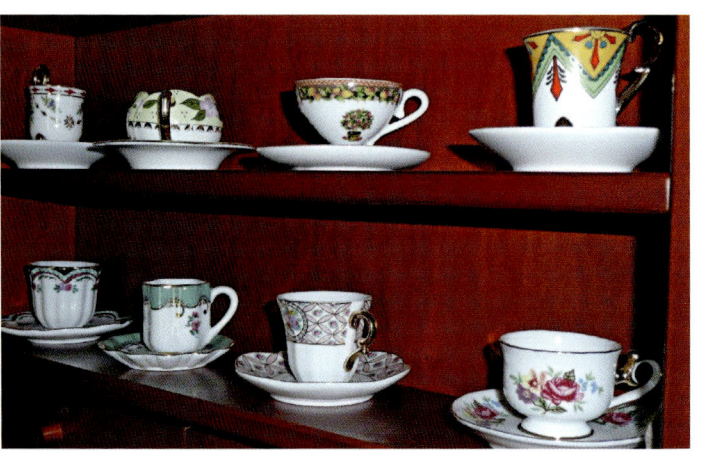

my collection of miniatures,

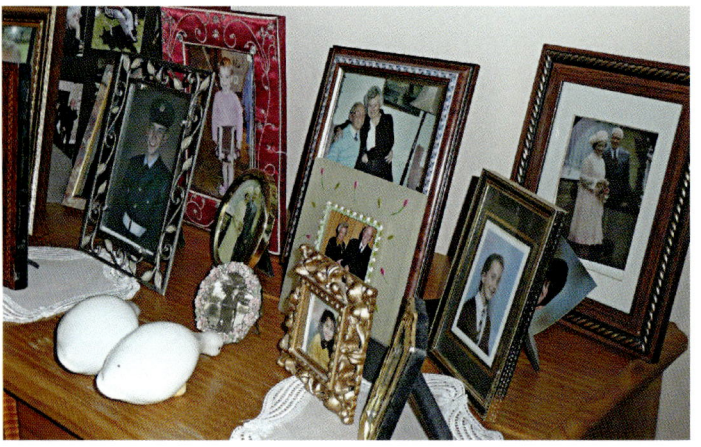

my pictures, photographs and ornaments.'

Special things from home are important for Gwen Morgan, so are her friends.

'In Burnham House I have got to know one or two people quite well. We have games and quizzes and I go on some of the trips. I have been to Westonbirt Arboretum and to a bird sanctuary. **I enjoy joining in some of the activities in the Day Centre.** I helped to decorate a pram for one of the flower competitions.

I have always been involved in the church and Bible groups so **I have made a lot of friends.** I used to live in Wales and some very good friends, who all go to the same church in Wales, come here to visit me.

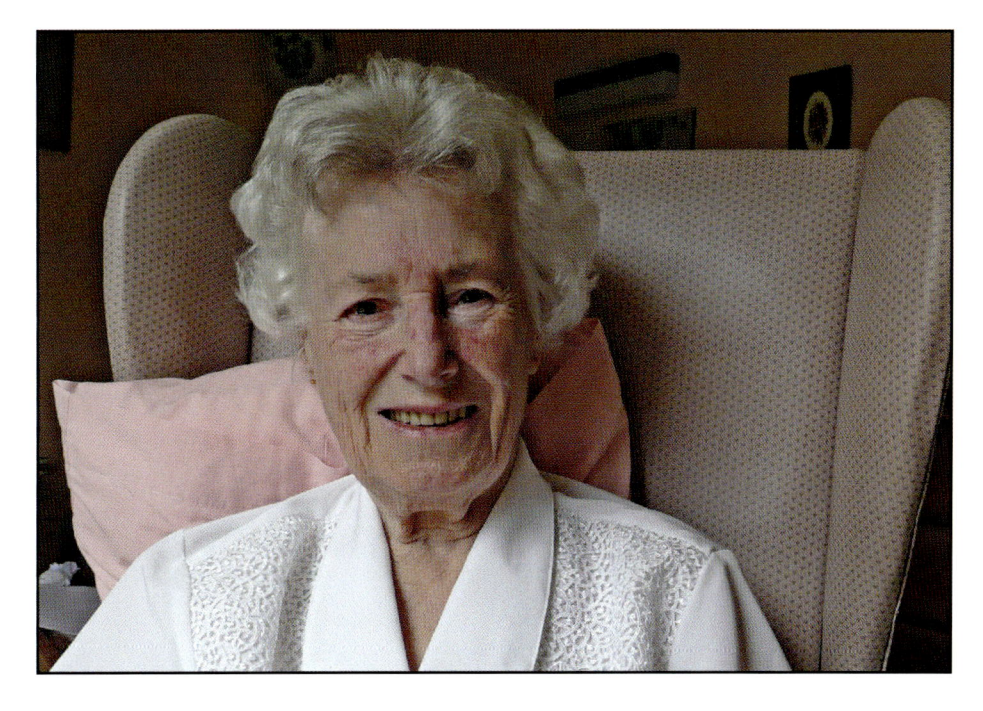

Gwen has always been involved in church and Bible groups

Now I feel I belong at Malmesbury Abbey, all my friends here are from the Abbey. I go to an Open Doors meeting every month. It is a chance to meet with people and have a beautiful lunch.
It is lovely to go into the countryside and meet up with my friends.

I like going out with my step son's wife, Margaret. She takes me for my beauty treatment, manicure and foot massage. I feel good afterwards.
I trained to be a secretary and worked for the Ministry of Agriculture during the war. There I met Howard who I married many years later.'

At the centre of Winnie's family tree is the photograph of her with her husband, Stanley, on their wedding day.
'When I have visits from my family, people spend a lot of time looking at the family tree and talking about it.' Muriel (Winnie) Miles

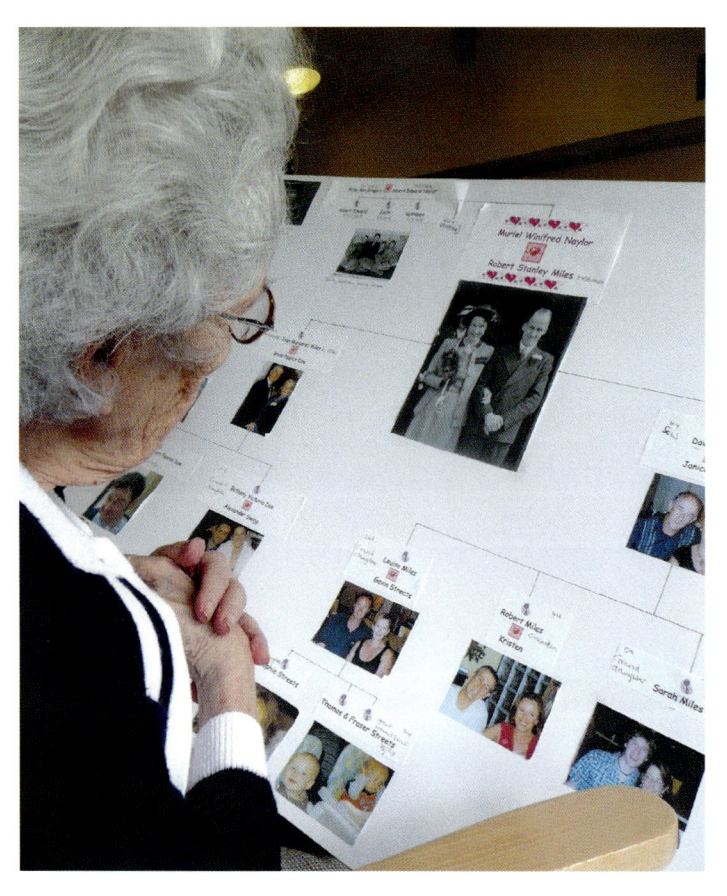

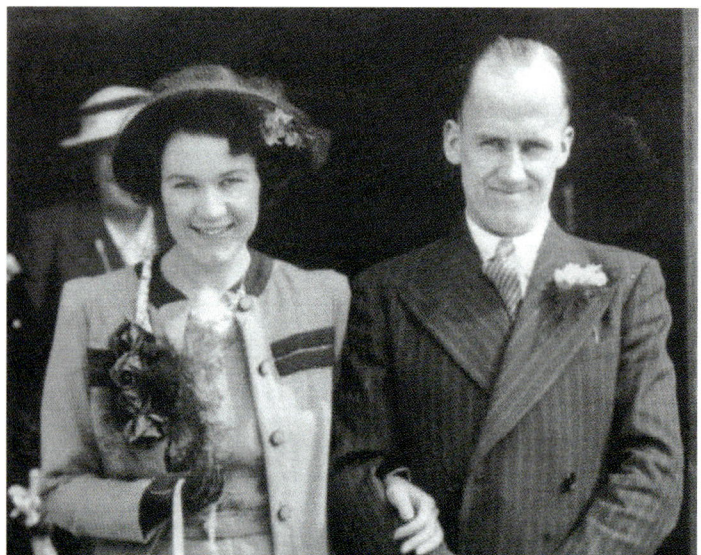

'People matter more than anything,' says Mary Bell

Mary loves to receive visits from her family. She and her husband, George, had six children and now she has fourteen grandchildren, eighteen great grandchildren and three great, great grandchildren!

'My family and people here have helped me to settle in. You get a lot of help.'

Mary served in World War II. *'I volunteered for the WAAFs when I was about nineteen years old. If you didn't volunteer for something you were conscripted. I worked in an office and I enjoyed it. We sent up the barrage balloons.*

My husband was in the Army. When the house where he lived got burned in an air raid, my brother brought him home to our house. That's how I met him. I've been extremely lucky. I did a lot of travelling abroad with George when he was a manager in a construction company. We even met the Queen twice!

It was much more romantic to travel in those days, not many people did. Actually it was unusual to be able to afford to travel, now more people do.

We lived in places like Jamaica and the Cayman Islands. There, we had maids to do the housework and nursery maids when we had the children.

I often think: did we really do this or that?'

Mary with great grand daughter Lucy.

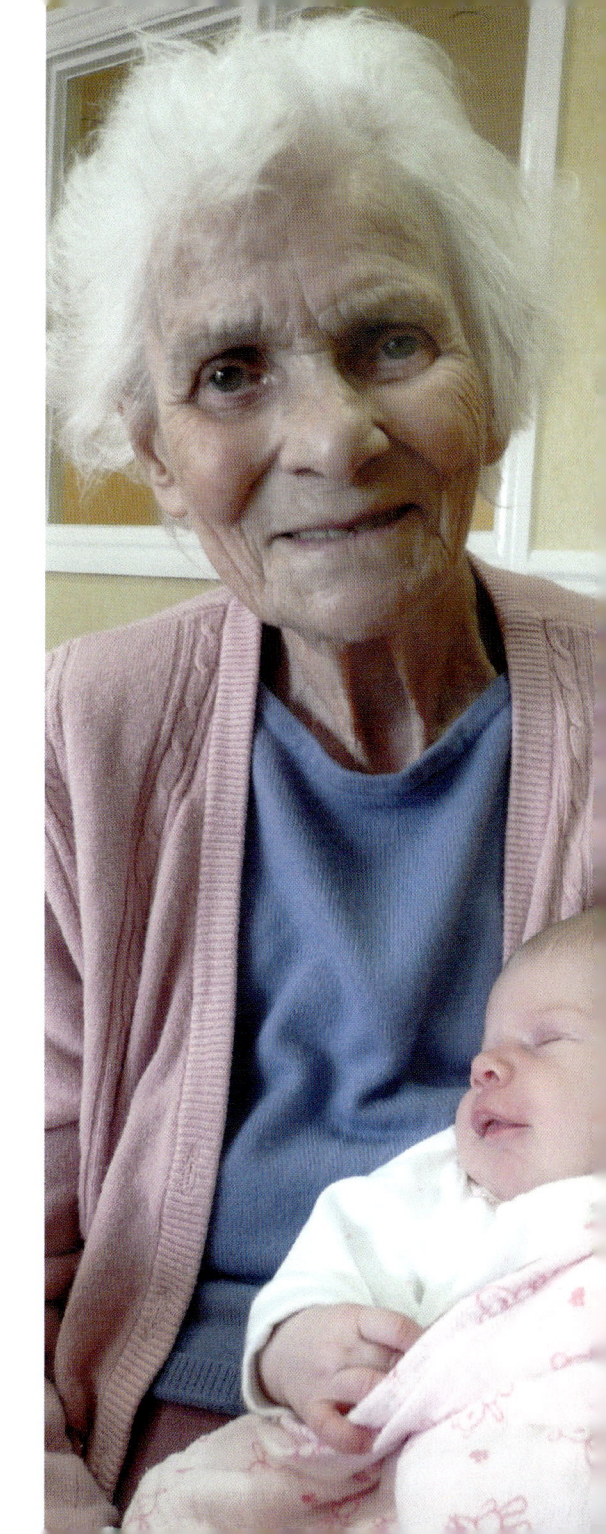

' It's a big thing to move from your house.'

Kathleen

35

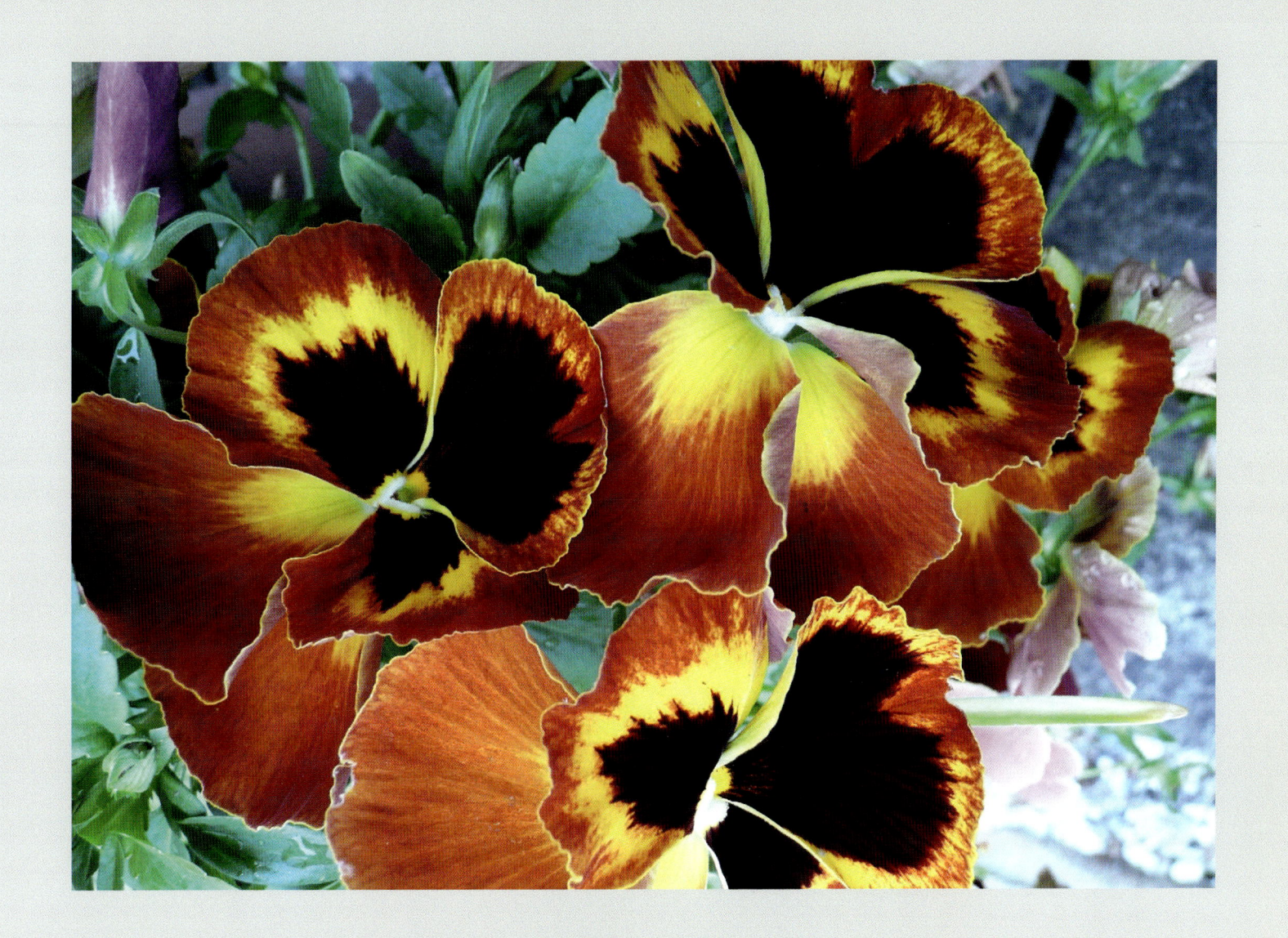

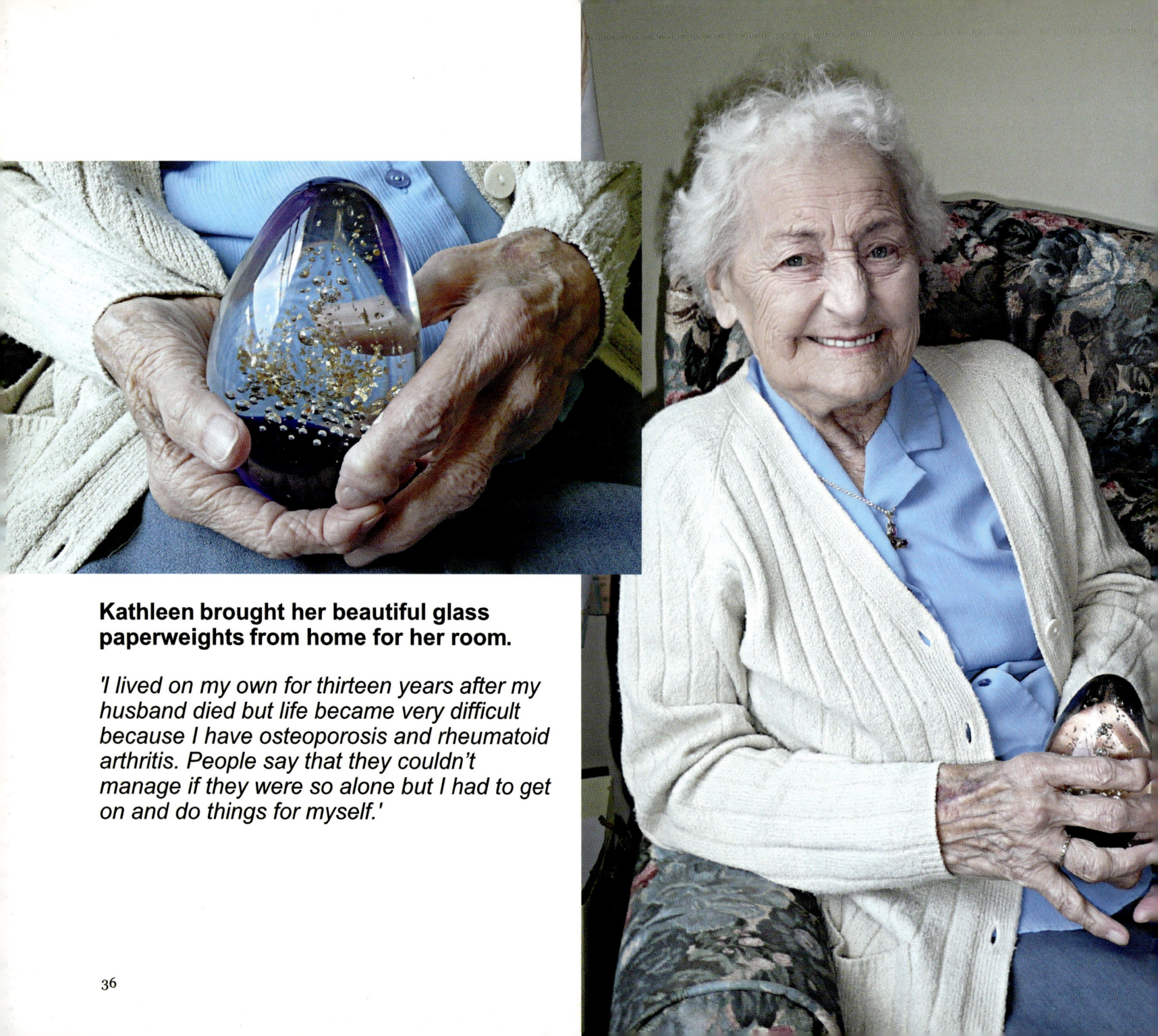

Kathleen brought her beautiful glass paperweights from home for her room.

'I lived on my own for thirteen years after my husband died but life became very difficult because I have osteoporosis and rheumatoid arthritis. People say that they couldn't manage if they were so alone but I had to get on and do things for myself.'

'I am the last member of my family. There is no-one from my twin brother's family living near but my nephew came from Canada to visit me when I was in intensive care after a fall.
When I came here I didn't know anyone, not a soul but now I have some friends.
In the morning I read in my room then after lunch I go to the Day Centre part of the lounge to be with company. After tea I like to watch television in my room.

When I was a teenager I couldn't go out as I pleased. I had to do everything in the house for half a crown a week. I did the washing for three beds, and the cooking. We didn't have a wringer.
I could wring the sheets and make them crack.

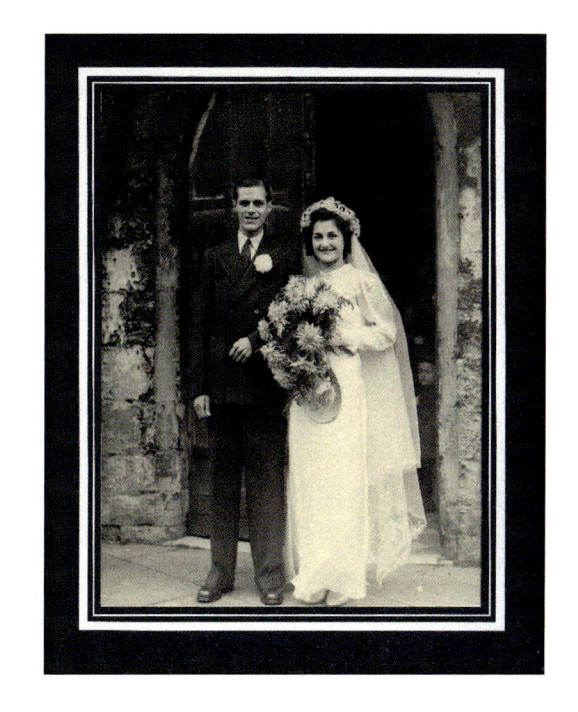

Kath and Frank were married in Chippenham Parish Church in 1944

Getting the boiler going and doing the washing was hard work. If I asked my mother how to do something she would say, "Find out". On a Sunday afternoon I'd be scrubbing the clothes ready for washing on Monday. My father worked on the boilers at Westinghouse. He was shovelling coal so his clothes got very dirty.
When I got married someone said, 'You are ever so lucky. Your initials spell KEPT, ***Kathleen Elsie Phyllis Tanner.'*** *We went to Weston-super-Mare for our honeymoon. Some people thought that we did not want children but we did; I cried. Nowadays you can get help.'*

Charles made his room a very personal space by bringing his desk and several, pieces of furniture from home. Also he has surrounded himself with an abundance of favourite pictures, family photographs, cartoons and other interesting mementos.

'I have newspapers everyday and enjoy doing the crossword puzzles. If I get stuck I can cry on the shoulders of my friends Peggy, Rosemary and Arthur who are very good at crossword puzzles and help me!
I enjoy reading and I write quite a lot of letters. I tend to pile books and papers around me when I am doing different things but it is not a problem here because this is my home.

I came here because my family thought that I was not looking after myself well enough. Actually they have been proved right. **Sometimes I think about having my own home again but weighing things up, it is better to be here with care, conversation and company.** *If I was on my own, with the responsibility of the home, garden and so on, it would be too difficult. I would miss the company and talking to people.'*

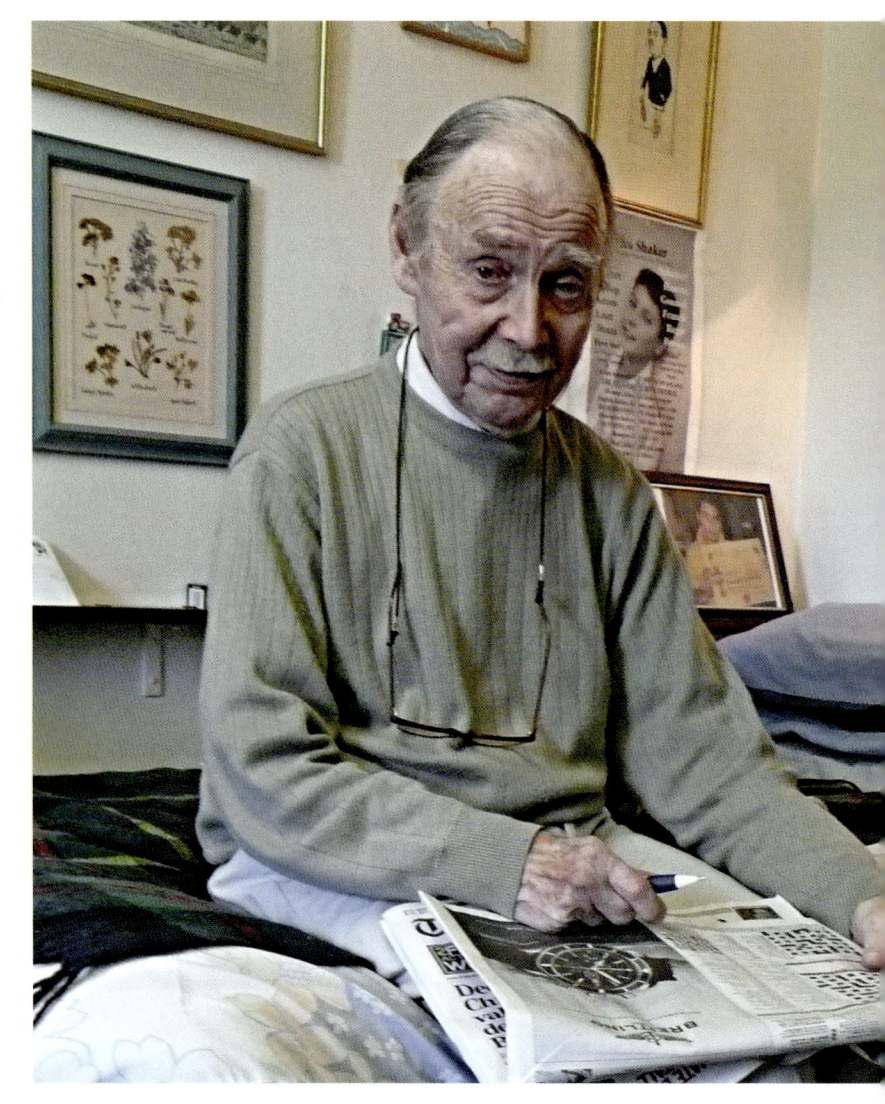

'I probably have more friends than relatives and have quite a few visitors. People are important and have always interested me as long as I know what they are saying. I was diagnosed as deaf when I was a few months old but with help from my mother and a doctor I learned to lip read.'

When Charles started work he had to choose between a career in brewing or munitions. He chose the brewing industry but later moved to the Stock Exchange.

'I had never really wanted to do brewing, I wanted something more exciting. The life, the people and the atmosphere in the Stock Exchange were wonderful.

It was useful to be able to lip read what the opposition was saying until they realised and started to say misleading information!

From my window I have a very good view of the flowerbed and garden where occasionally I see a fox.

The photographs of my wife, Gilly, and my brother are particularly important to me. My wife gave me something that no other lady could give me.

The baronetcy came to me from my paternal grand father after the death of my brother in the 1943 Battle of Salerno.'

Sir Charles Mcleod, Bt

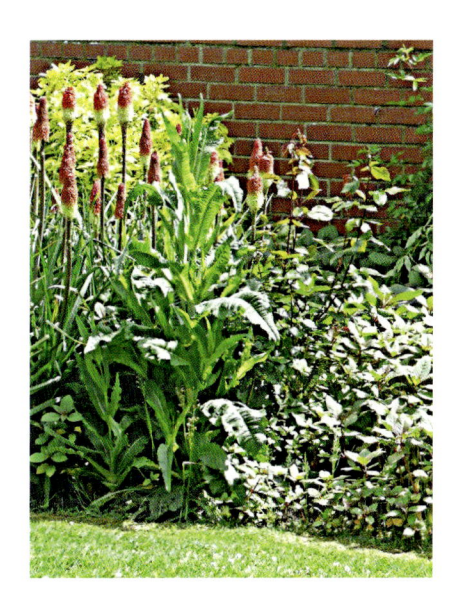

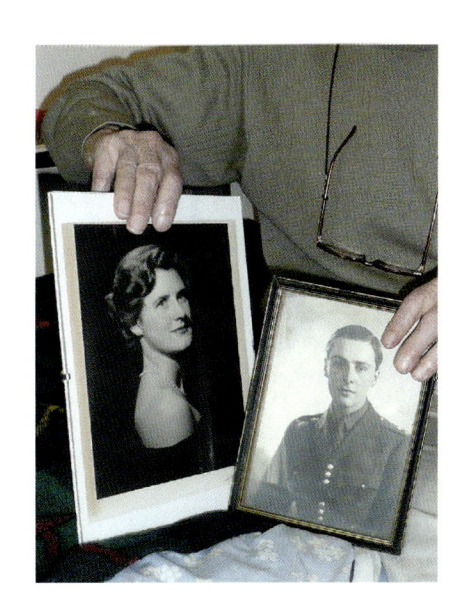

39

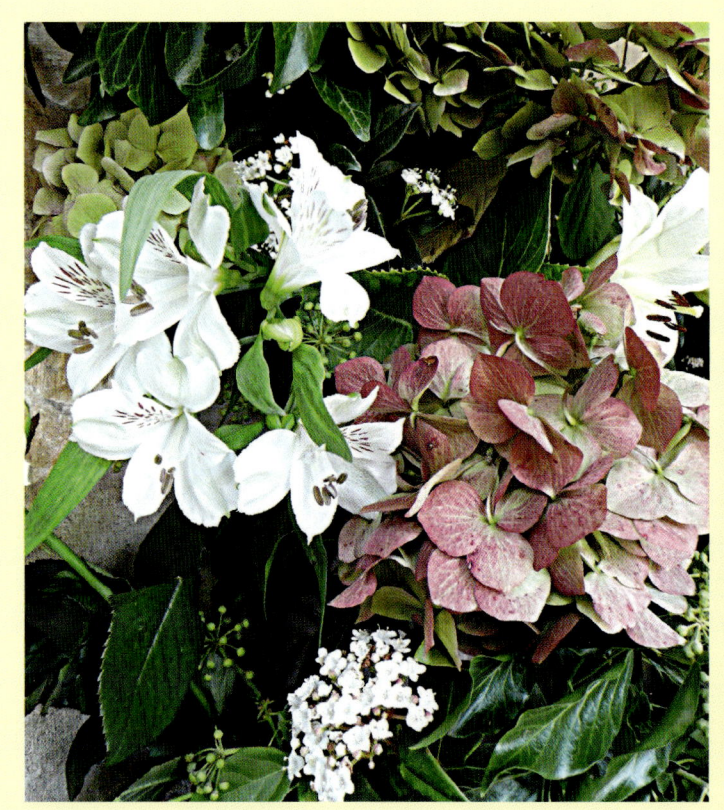

'The only things I can remember queuing up for during the war were bananas.'

Bertha

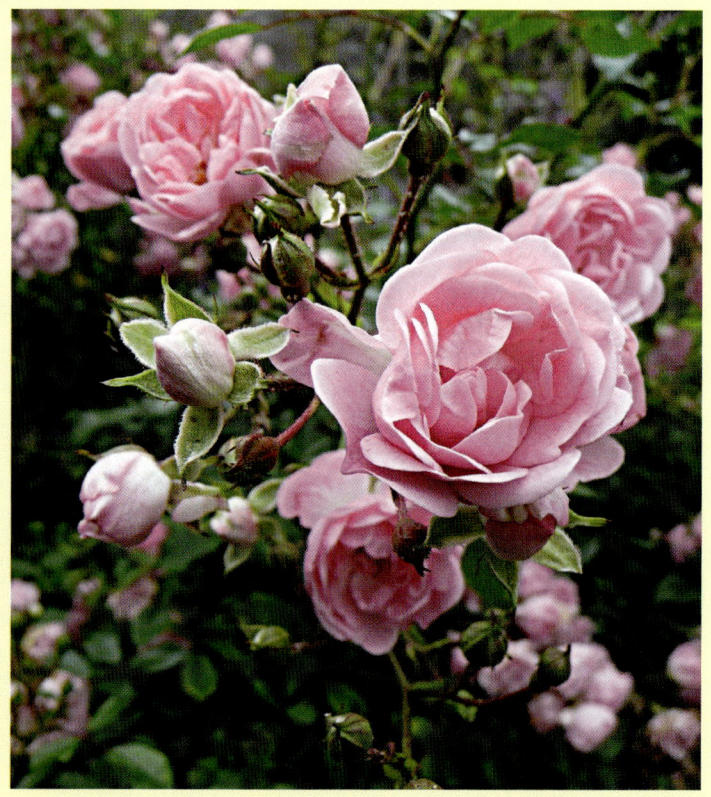

'I queued up for everything.'

Queenie

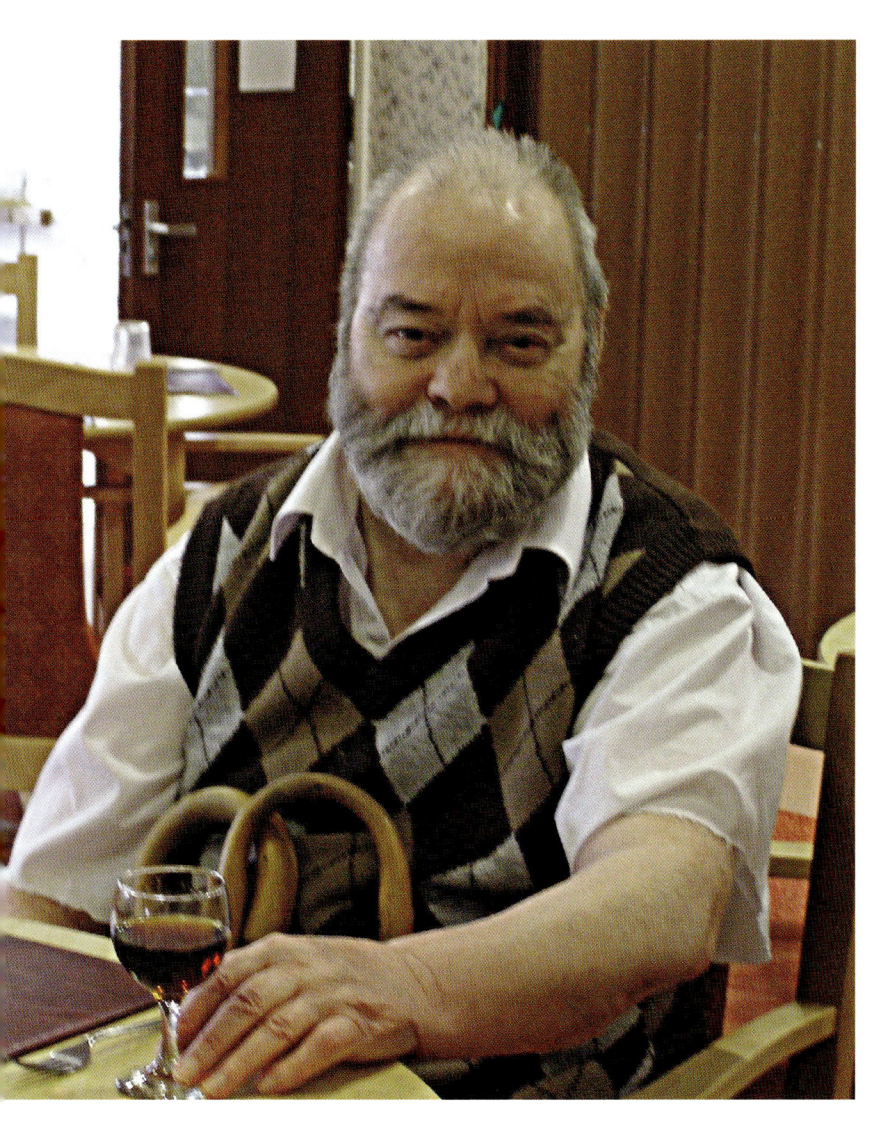

Time with friends is important for Ken

'In the morning I like to be downstairs so that I can talk to my friends. Every day my friend James and I meet in the dining room for a drink before lunch. I usually have a glass of sherry and James has a glass of French wine.

Originally I came from Liverpool. I joined up in 1942 when I was eighteen years old. **I was on an LCM** (Landing Craft Mechanised) **during the D-day landings in Northern France.** We carried the Eighth Army soldiers who had come from the desert. We waded in the water and made a human chain to rescue the Americans shot down over Normandy. I have three medals for my service in the Royal Marines.

After I was "demobbed" I spent forty years on the road and walked thousands of miles as a "gentleman of the road". I walked the length and breadth of England, Scotland and Wales. **Like Frank Sinatra, "I did it my way".** All that walking took its toll and I had to have a hip replacement operation.'

Ken Hudson

Bertha had a busy life bringing up six children. It is no wonder that she enjoys being with people and having visitors.

'I'm happy enough. I like company. It is lovely when you meet with people you have met before.

I like going on little outings.

I have always loved singing and I love singing my hymns. I used to sing every Sunday in church. When I was in the WAAFs we used to go into hospitals and sing to the patients.'

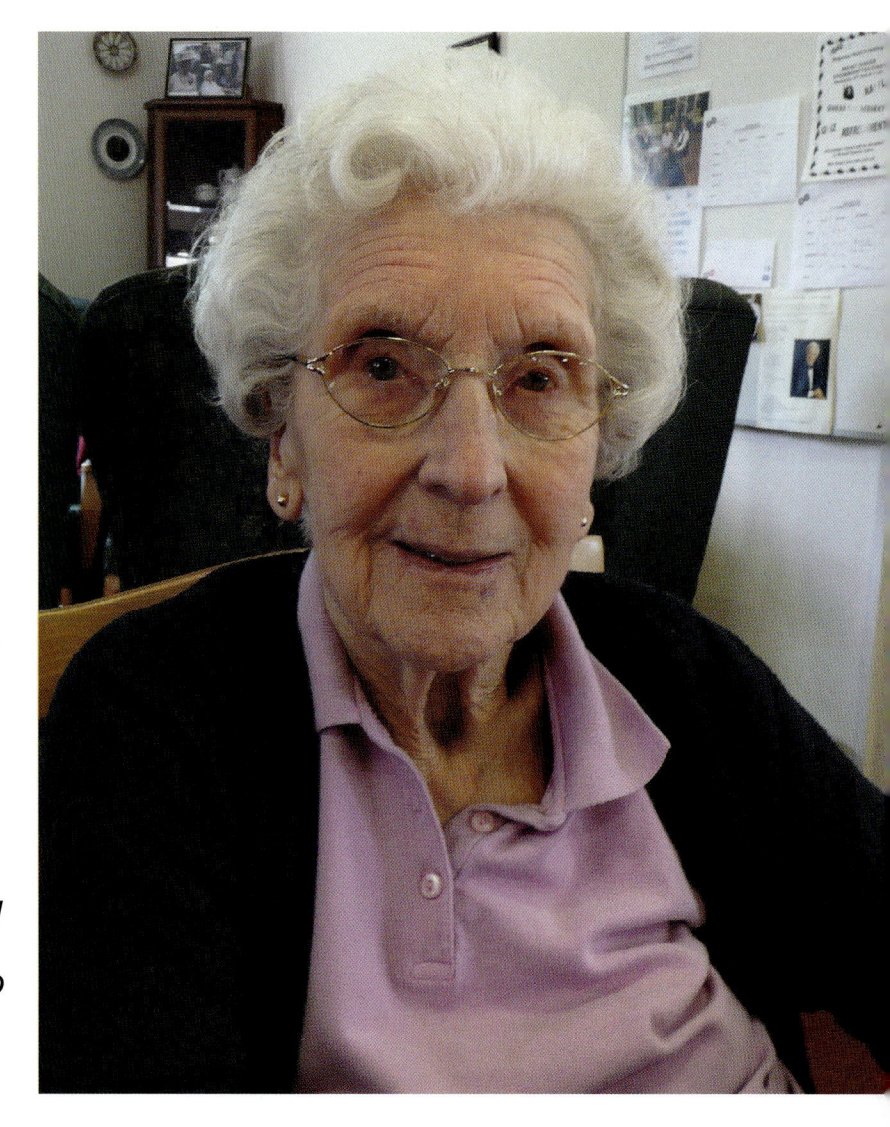

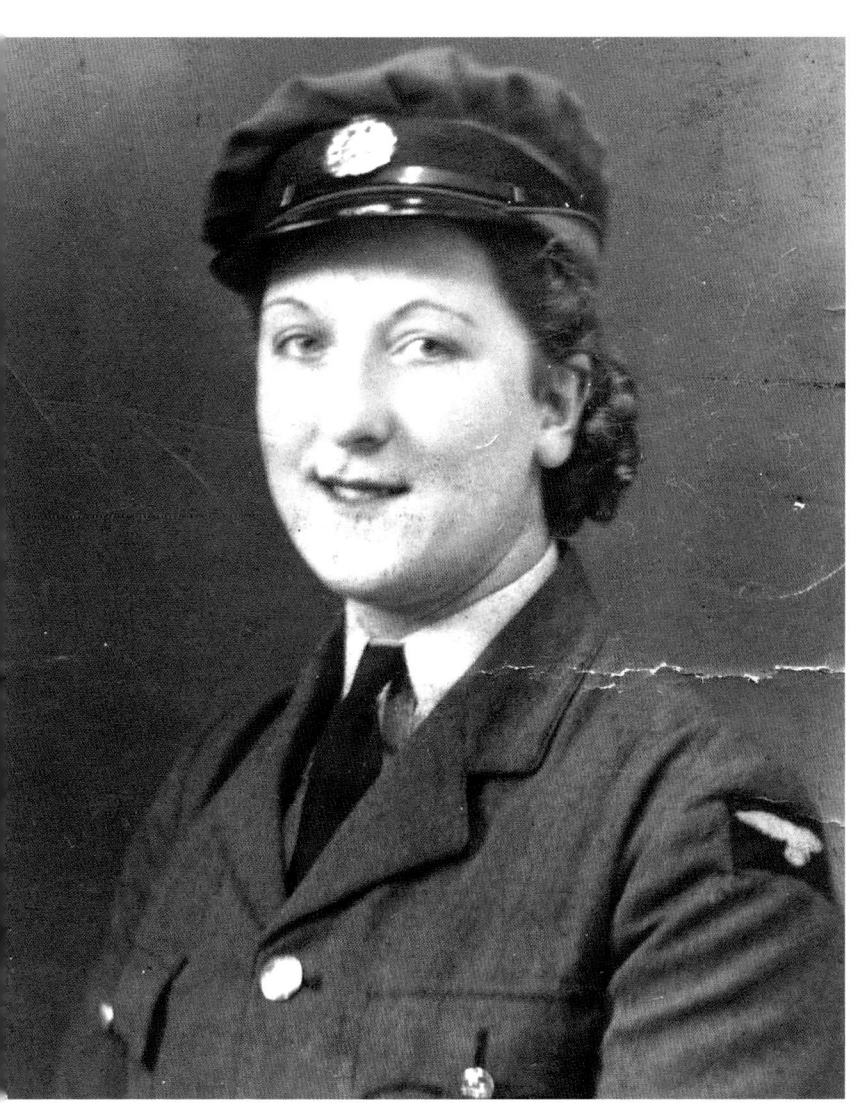

Bertha volunteered to join the Women's Auxilliary Air Force in 1942 when she was twenty years old. She served in Melksham and Edgehill.

'When I was in the WAAFs I was an L.A.C. (Leading Air Craft woman).
I did the cooking but not for long. I always remember when we had to make huge pans of soup. You had to chop all those vegetables!

I liked the uniform but hated going out in uniform, especially if you passed an officer. You had to stand to attention and salute.

I met my husband when he was in the Royal Air Force. He said to me,

"I'm going to keep my eye on you."

He kept getting himself put on "jankers" so that he could see me in the kitchen. Sometimes he had to wash the cooking tins.'

Some of Bertha's memories of her time in the WAAFs were shared in a Remembrance Day service in her village church at Lea in 2006.

Do you have a favourite place here?

'I like being down in the lounge with company, we talk to each other. I could do a lot more if I didn't have to use a walking frame.

When I first came here I came everyday to the Day Centre, it was lovely.

Doing things is better than doing nothing. We do exercises in our chairs, ball games and other things. I enjoy going on trips but it's difficult to get out with my walker.

I love to see the family but my granddaughters live in London. My grandson, Jonathan, is lovely. He came to see me on my birthday.'

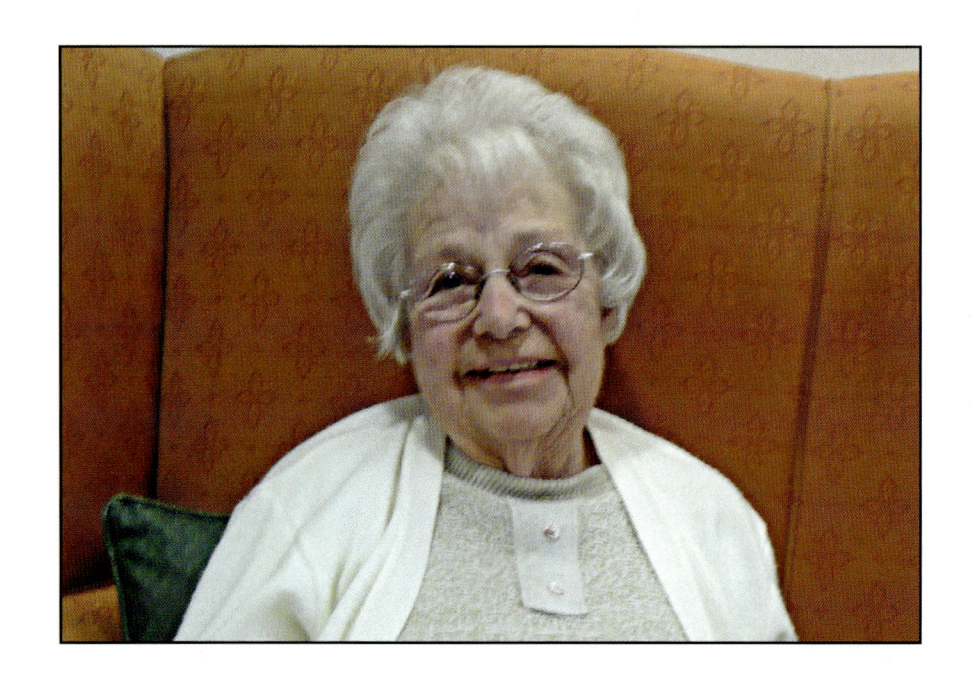

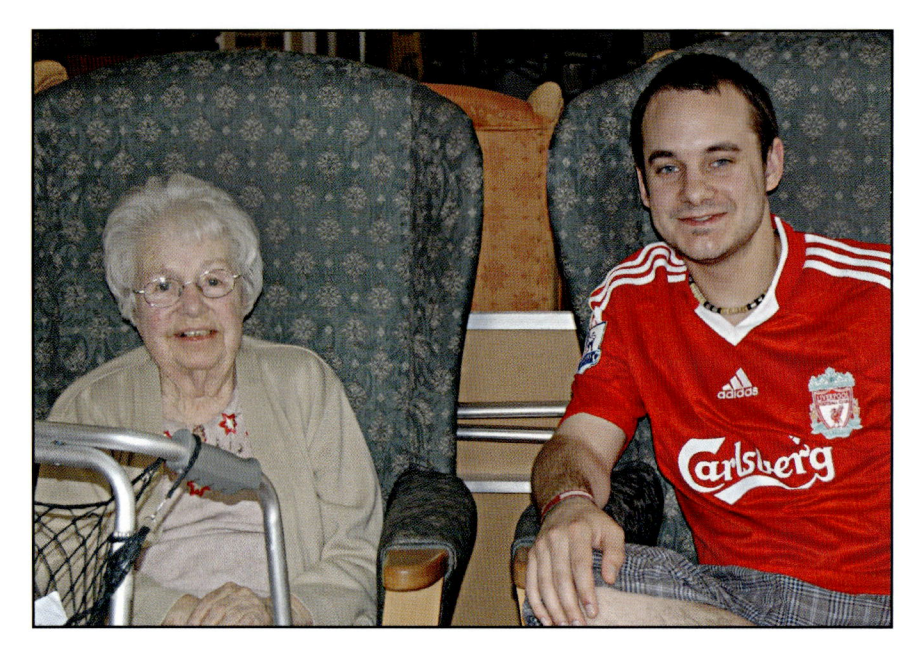

Jonathan with Elsie on her 90th birthday. Photo by Keith Sharpe

'When I left school I was fourteen. My mother was not well. There were five children. I was the eldest and she wanted me to stay at home to look after the family. In the end I retaliated and said,
"Look I'm not doing this all the time."
In the end I went to do hairdressing. I was mad on it. I helped the hairdresser do perms and **I took to the haircutting very quickly.** You got tips but not everybody gave them, maybe a sixpence or a threepenny bit. A shilling would be a lot.

One day in the war, when I got off the bus to go to work, a policeman stopped me to ask,
"Where are you going?"
"I'm going up there to the hairdressers; I work there."
He said, **"You won't be able to work there any more, it has been bombed."**
Later the butcher's wife set up a hairdresser's shop and I ran it for her. One of my hairdressing customers asked me if I would do her hair at her home at night so I said I would. She said,

"Don't be surprised if you see two young men. I agreed to have them as lodgers."
When I had finished doing her hair both of these fellows said that they would walk me home because it was dark. **They argued a bit and I let them but Jack Sharpe won.** I married Jack, a wonderful man.'

Elsie Sharpe

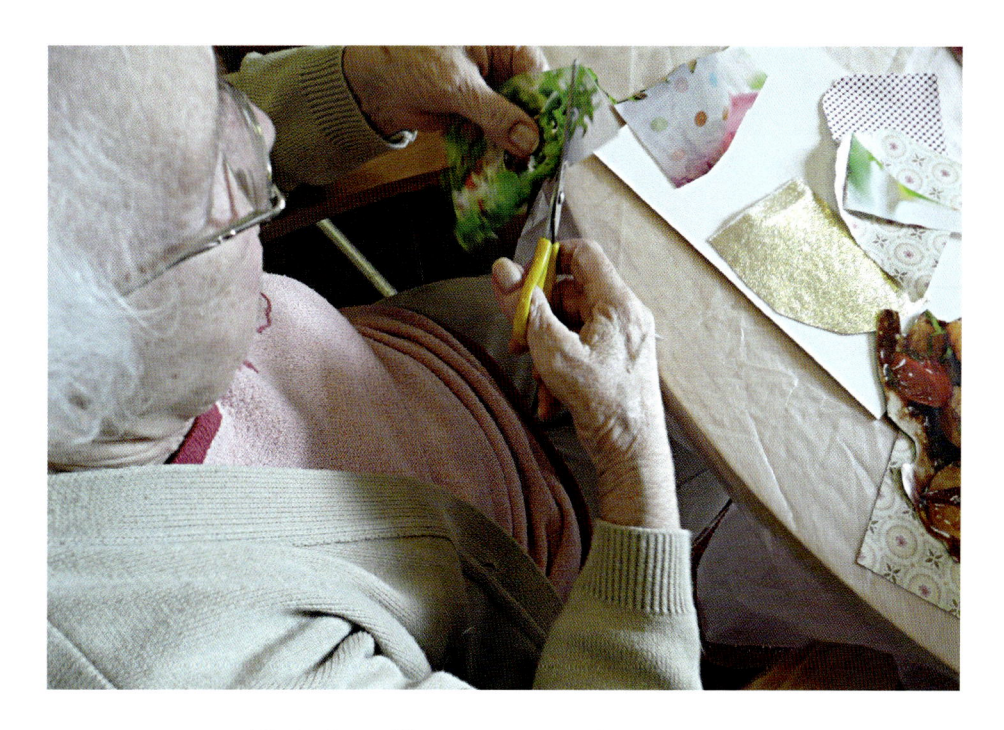

Elsie is still an expert with scissors

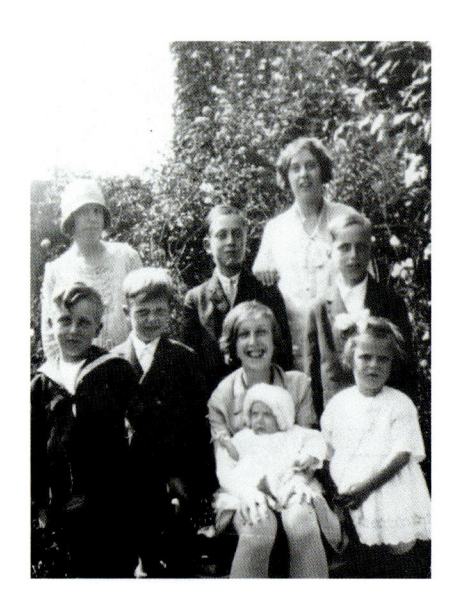

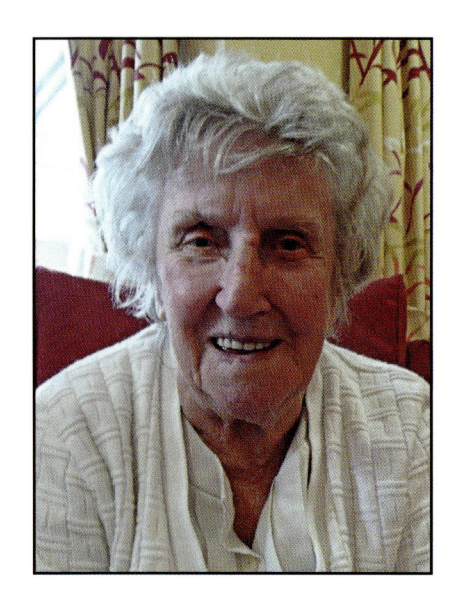

Marie loves being in company

Maybe it is not surprising that Marie loves being with people because she is used to the company of a large family.

In this family photograph Marie, holding her baby sister, is with her eight brothers and sisters.

Marie can remember her father selling fresh fish from his donkey and cart that he took around Bournemouth before World War Two.

Marie worked as a housekeeper when she was younger. Now she likes to go on outings or spend time in the lounge where she takes an active part in some of the activities.
'I like being with people and I like singing.'
Marie Bailey

Marie had a lucky escape during the war.
In September 1940 Marie's husband was serving in the Army in Germany when their house in Croydon was bombed. Marie was sleeping under the stairs during the bombing and was buried under the debris. People heard her shouting so she was rescued and taken to hospital. A badly broken leg kept her in hospital for four months. Her son, Brian, still has the telegram that informed his father of the disaster. They received £110.00 compensation for the loss of their home.

A newspaper report shows that all the rooms were shattered but the mirror over the fireplace in the bedroom was unbroken! A remarkable piece of good luck, perhaps?

Hetty really enjoyed her life in the WRNS

Hetty has been living in Burnham House for only a short while. She loves meeting people but says,
'I wouldn't say "Boo" when I was a child. Now, my speech is not very good. I keep losing my place.'

Hetty has some happy memories of her war service in Bournemouth.

'I used to work in Customs and Excise before the war. Then I was in the WRNS. It was wonderful. It was part of my life that I really enjoyed, some of the happiest days of my life. I put on weight when I was in the WRNS because I was so happy. **We called the office I worked in "The Ship" but I never went to sea on a ship while I was in the WRNS!** I used to cycle from my billet to "The Ship" but when we went to dances the bus that took us was a three ton lorry that we called the "Liberty Boat"!
I met my husband when he was in the RAF. He was tall, over six foot, blonde and a very good looking chap'.

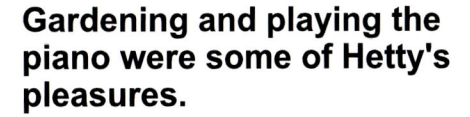

Gardening and playing the piano were some of Hetty's pleasures.

'I love the air and fields and grass.

I loved playing the piano; I played by ear but couldn't read music. I used to play in my grandfather's piano shop. The children used to watch and listen to me through the window.'

Hetty Weatherley

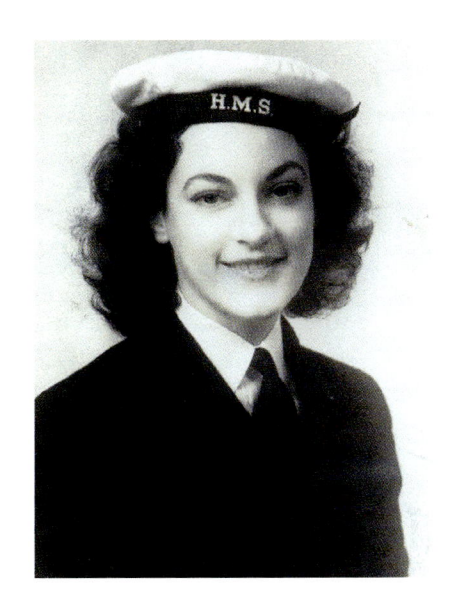

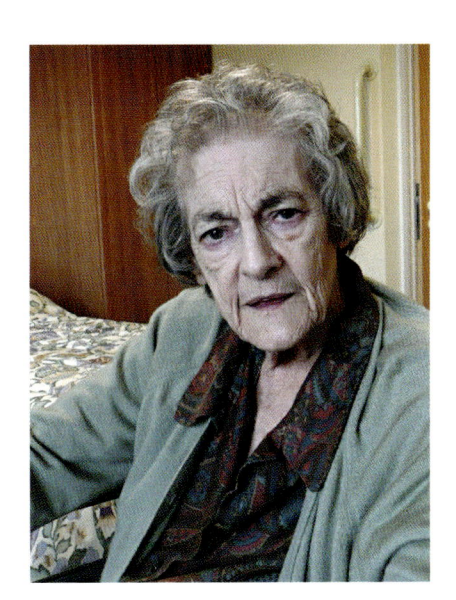

The sound of music can often be heard drifting from Arthur's room

'I spend a lot of my time in my room but I'm not bored or lonely. I enjoy listening to music. My daughter chose my bookcase and the music centre cabinet from my flat to bring here for me. My cabinet came with all my tapes and CDs, mostly 1930s and 1940s music by people like Al Bowlly, Bing Crosby, Dean Martin and Perry Como. I like American Sweet Bands and singers like Patsy Cline and Dorothy Squires. I like some classical music too.'

Arthur is a regular listener to BBC Radio Wiltshire at weekends when, in the evenings, David Lowe plays just the kind of music and songs from the 1920s to the 1950s that Arthur enjoys.

'In the afternoons I watch television programmes like "Countdown" and I watch some of the "soaps". Sometimes I go out on the day trips and my daughter visits me and takes me out too. **I like to do tapestry work. This tapestry could be for a fire screen.***'*

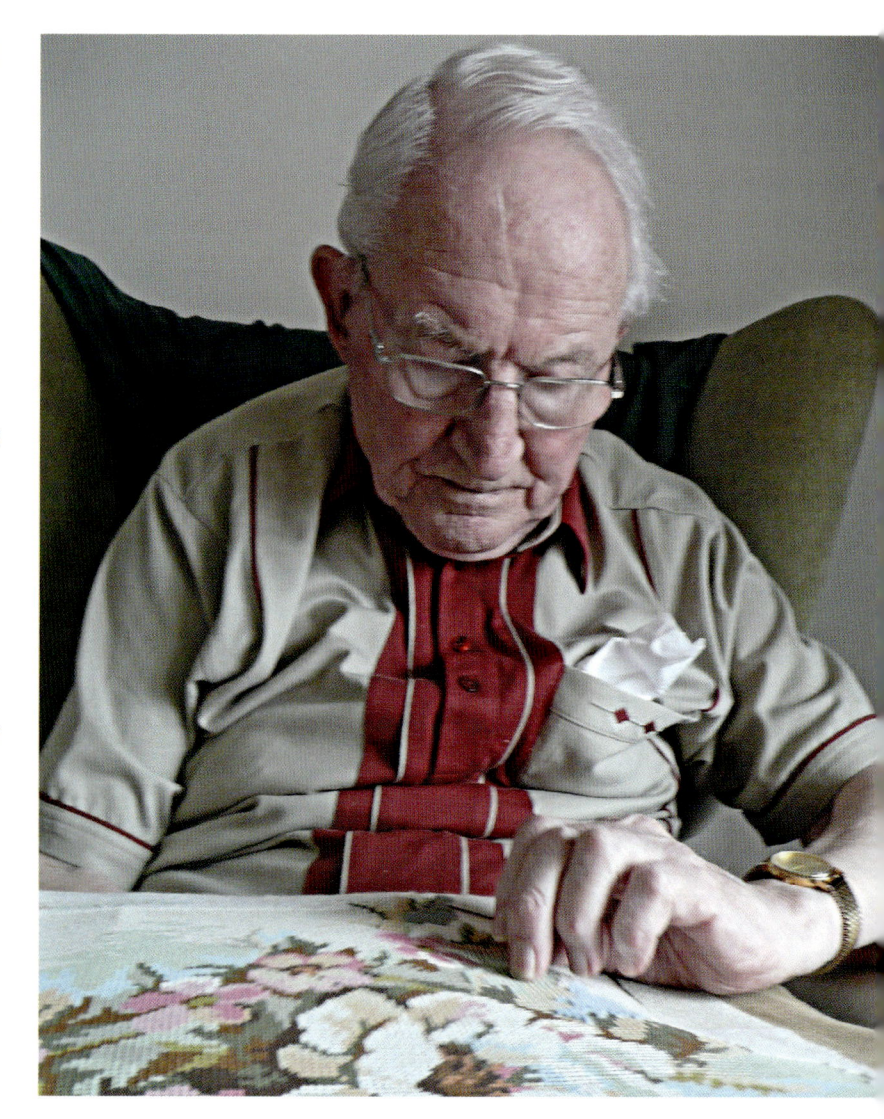

'In 1946, after the end of the war, when I was in the Army in Germany, I injured my ankle very badly when I was playing rugby against an RAF team that had come out from England. After the operation on my ankle I went to an Army rehabilitation centre. In the centre you had your treatment and then for the rest of the day you did what you wanted to but they didn't like to see you doing nothing. That's when I started to do tapestry work. I made a firescreen and I still have it today. You could buy your materials there and I taught myself although there was a lady in charge who could help. I have been doing tapestry work on and off ever since. I have made pictures and I have made kneelers for churches. One kneeler is in the church at Hankerton.'

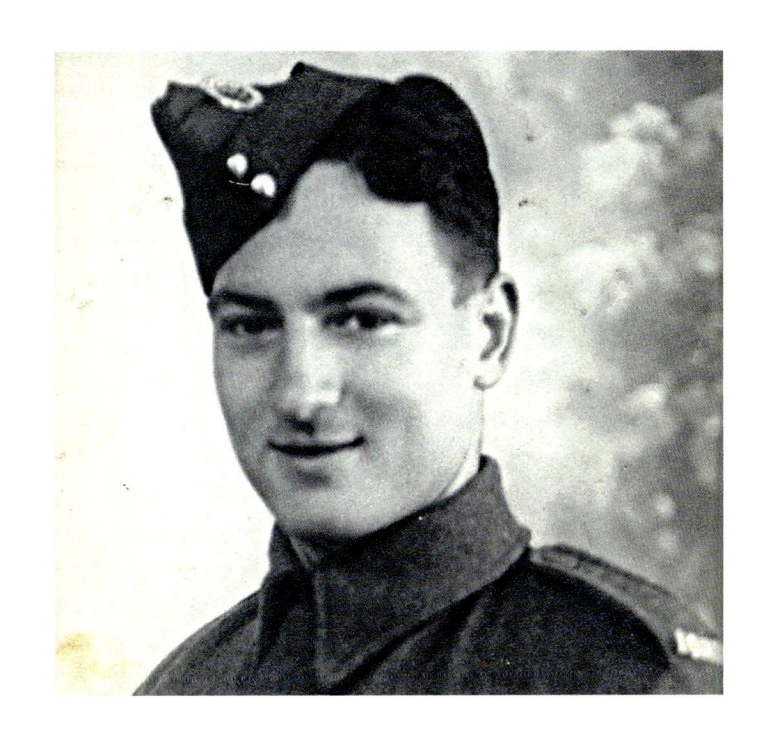

Eighteen year old Arthur Blott was called up in 1943

What did you do while you were in the Army?

'I remember hearing Neville Chamberlain announcing that we were going to be at war. I was at home doing my homework. No-one thought that the war would last as long as it did, six years. When I was called up I went to Prestatyn first but then I went all over the place to different aerodromes. I was a signals operator working with keyboards and line, morse code and teleprinters. We didn't go abroad until 1944 when we went to Normandy. We were in the Air Formation Signals attached to the Spitfire squadron pilots and the Free French pilots.'

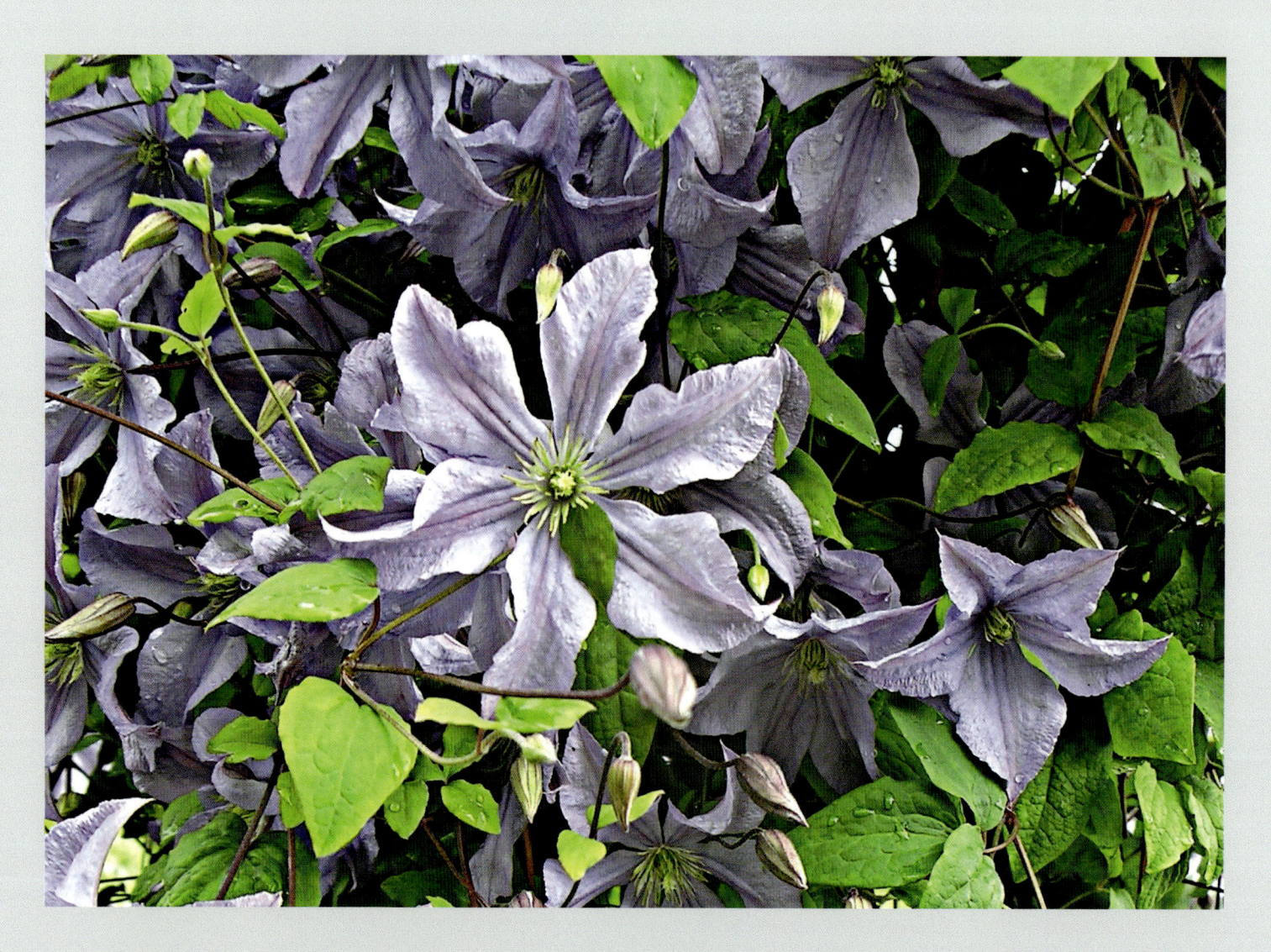

'Doing something is much better than doing nothing.'

Elsie

A 1950s Tea Dance - in costume! **A collage workshop**

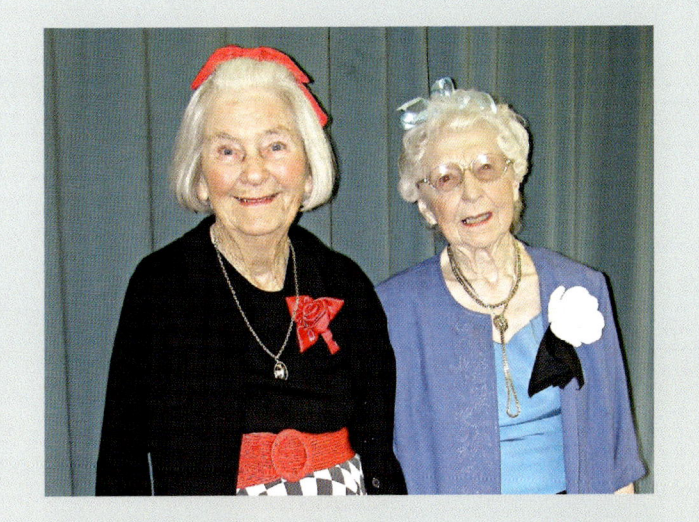

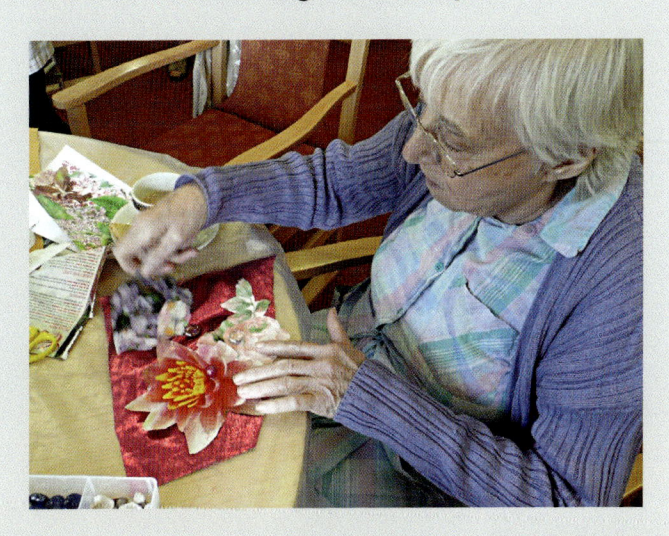

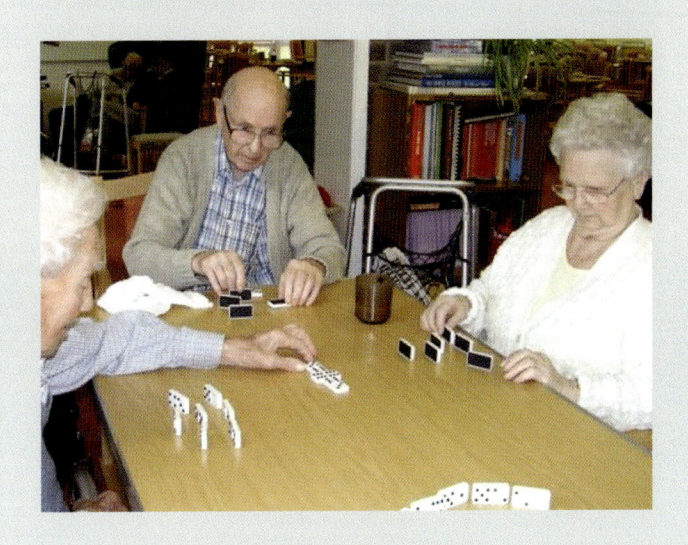

A game of dominoes **Drawing and painting**

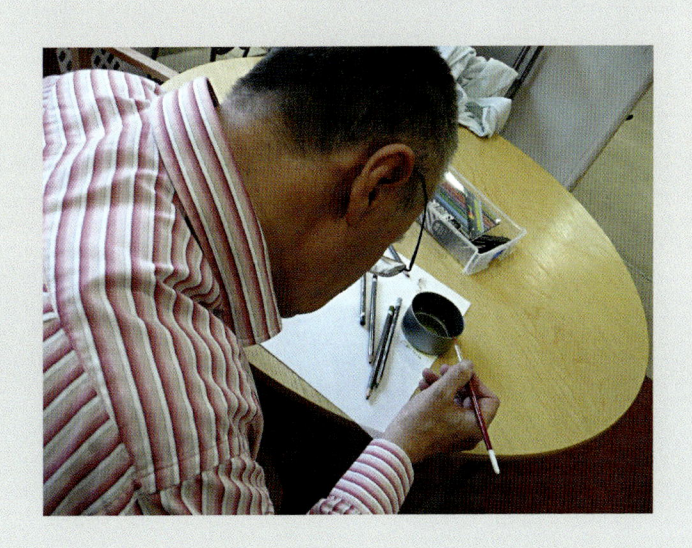

As a hotel manager James became very used to making a new home in different places. He has made his room his own with his desk and some of the Copenhagen ceramics that he and his wife Betty collected, as well as many pictures, mementos and photographs of their travels.

James and his wife grew up together because their mothers were friends who lived in the same street in Paisley and sang in the same choir. The families went on holiday together too. James went to college near Glasgow to train in hotel management and for many years, after his marriage to Betty, they lived in the hotels that he managed.

Sadly, James and Betty had to move from their house in Trowbridge after James had a heart attack and Betty developed Alzheimer's disease.

'Betty has moved to Chippenham now so I am able to visit her regularly every week. Here I enjoy talking to people and going out, especially with my daughter and son-in-law who live and work in London. They took me on the London Eye for my eightieth birthday.'

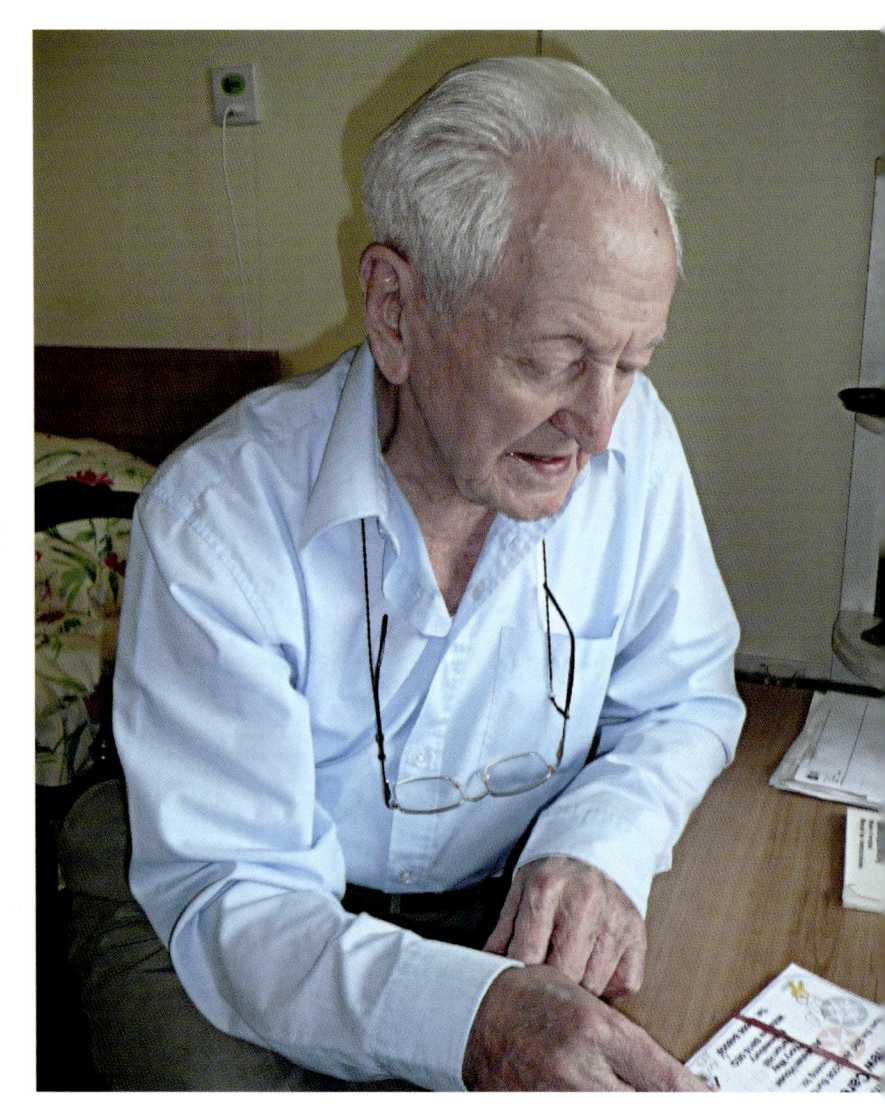

'When I am in my room I listen to the radio or music on my CD player. Before lunch I like to go to the dining room to have a glass of wine with my friend, Ken.

I enjoy watching sport on the television.
We had a nice evening in my room watching a football final. It started when Sid said that what he would really like is some champagne and caviar. Sid, Bill, Arthur and I sorted out an event worth celebrating. We thought that the UEFA Champions League final was a good occasion. **We had caviar on melba toast, onion cheese spread on little biscuits and champagne.** *It was a very nice night. I was happy to see Manchester United win. The manager is a Scot like me.*

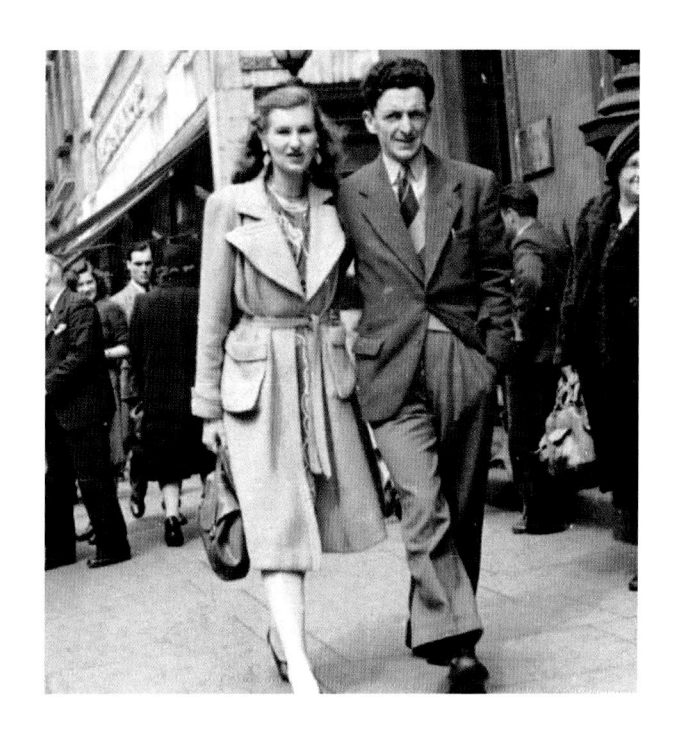

James and Betty on their honeymoon in 1947

I worked as an assistant manager or manager in four and five star hotels in places such as Stratford-upon-Avon, Edinburgh, Oban and Harrogate. I am used to meeting all kinds of people. I dealt with royalty, prime ministers and film stars like Bob Hope, Bing Crosby and Katherine Hepburn.

Betty and I used to enjoy our holidays abroad. When we stayed in hotels and went into the dining room my wife would say,
"You sit there."
I had to sit with my back to the room so that I couldn't see what the waiters and staff were doing!'

James Clark

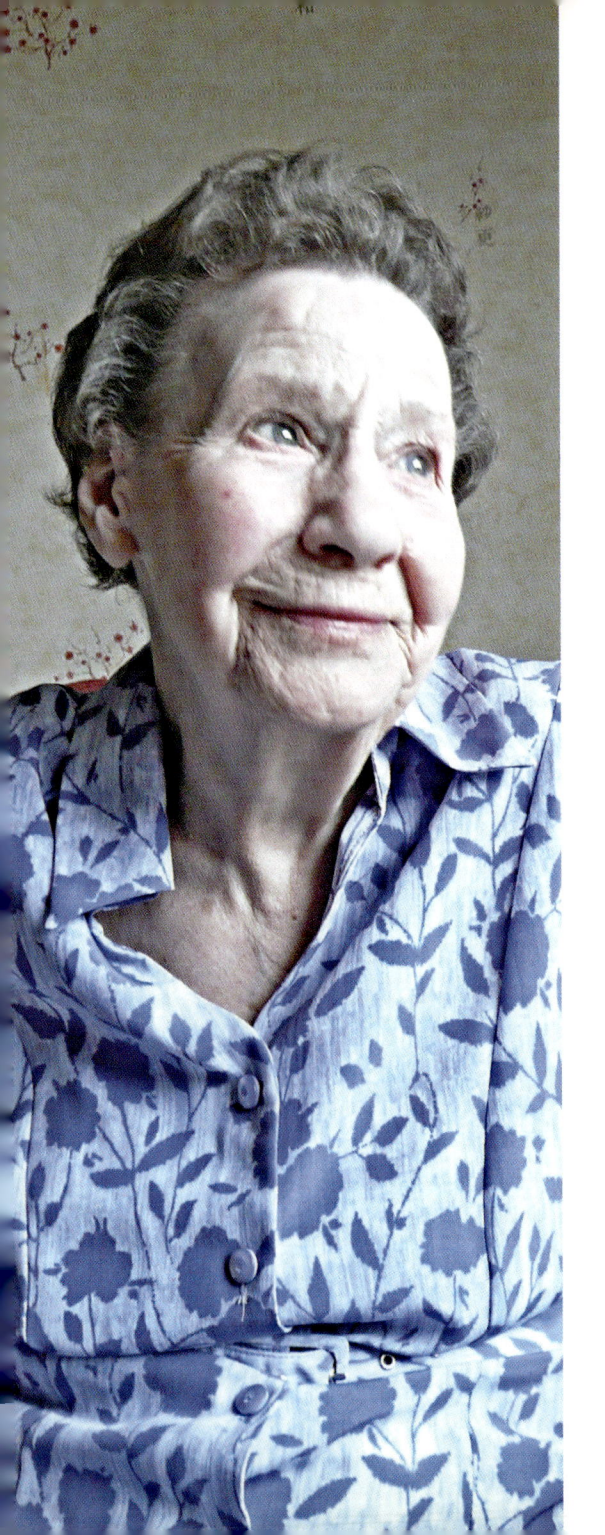

Phyllis and George Elms are pleased to be together

'**Before we came to Burnham House George and I were both ill but we didn't want to be parted. We asked if we could both come here and we have rooms next to each other.**

I have photographs and chairs from home and I have a lamp that George converted from a vase. It was important for me to be able to bring my own reclining armchair for my room.

I need quiet time every day and usually spend the morning in my room. I don't want to be there all of the time but I enjoy spending some time in my own room. For instance I like to go there to watch the television news after tea. I like to keep in touch with current affairs and the outside world.

I love reading and I read in my room because I can't concentrate downstairs in the lounge. I've always belonged to the library ever since I can remember.

I love going out with my daughter Penny and my grandsons. They are very good to me. **We go out into the "normal" world and I feel that I am recapturing a bit of the life I used to have.**

I look forward to going to the Luncheon Club in Malmesbury Town Hall. The WRVS cook the lunches. They are lovely meals, beautifully presented.

I enjoy playing skittles and I like quizzes. We go to other Homes to do things like bingo and darts. I got to the semi-finals in the darts competition.'

Phyllis remembers meeting George for the first time.

*'I first saw him in the canteen at Ekco where we worked. I was going out with another young man at the time but then George asked me for a date. I told him,
"You will have to find where to come".
He found me and brought a box of Black Magic chocolates.* **I thought he wasn't bad looking and he had expectations.** *It was a long time before I brought him home. Malmesbury was like a village then but George came from Chippenham so my father thought he was a foreigner. My father was a nature loving man who liked crayfishing and rabbiting. George did the same in Chippenham so they got on very well together. George used to cycle to Malmesbury to take me home to his mum for tea. Then he used to take me home and have to cycle back to Chippenham!'*

During the war Phyllis worked at the Ekco factory as a winder in the Coil Shop. There was a bonus scheme for fast workers and Phyllis was one of them. Her prize was a visit to Bristol to go aboard a Destroyer.

George's war service was spent on the continent in the Signals Regiment. He joined Ekco after the war and ran the Model Shop.

Phyllis and George inherited ancient rights granted in 939 by King Athelstan to the Commoners of Malmesbury.

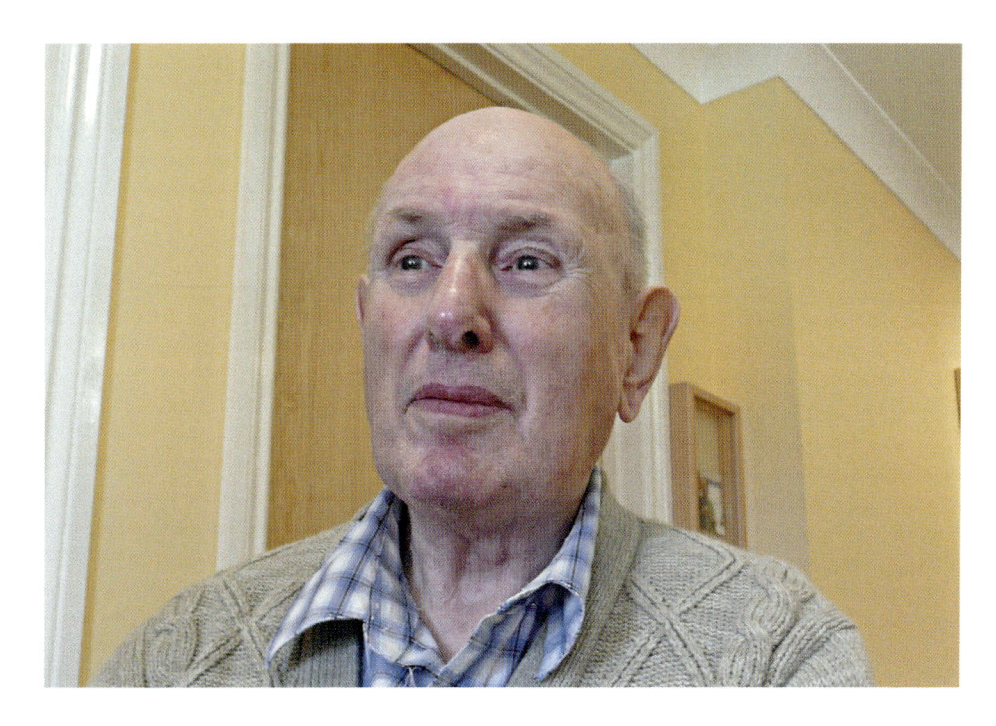

George is a Capital Burgess of the Borough of Malmesbury

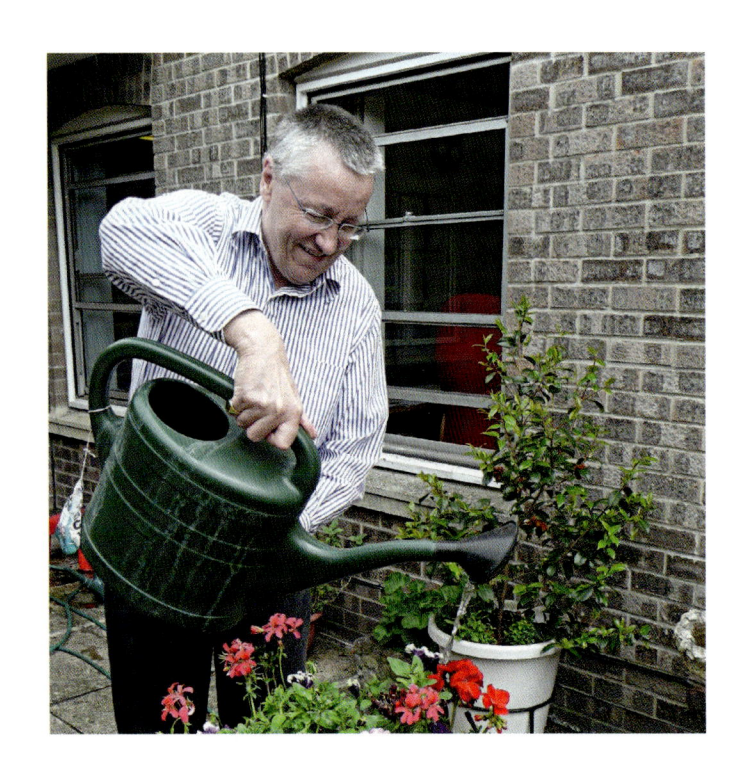

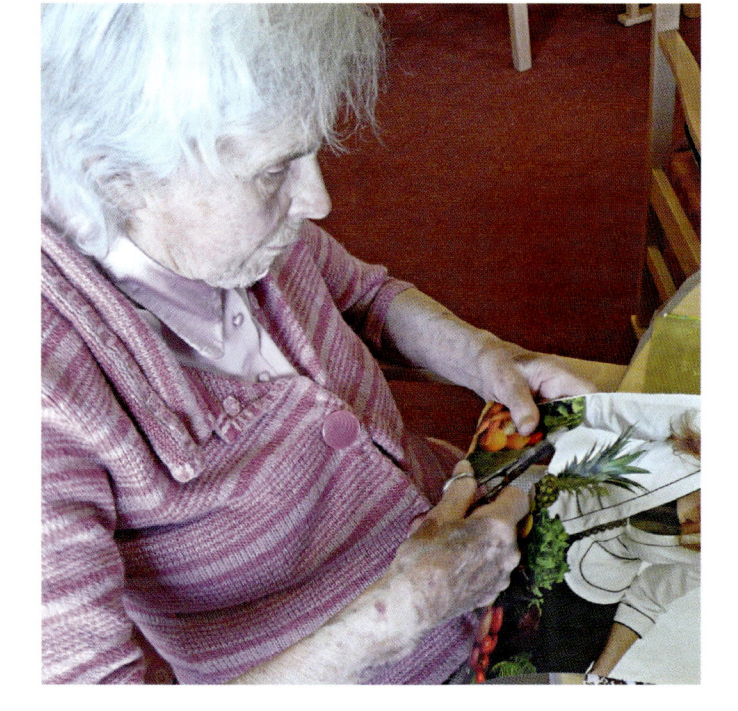

'I like going out, not just for the sake of it but to see or do something challenging. I went on several camps when I was a Scout leader. Four of us went camping last year. It was horrible weather but we stuck it out. I like to be with people and do things.'
Geoffrey Richardson

Betty used to be a junior school teacher. Her practical skills and sense of colour and design are assets in the art workshops.
'I like to spend some time with other people and be where I can join in some of the things that are going on.'
Betty Parsons

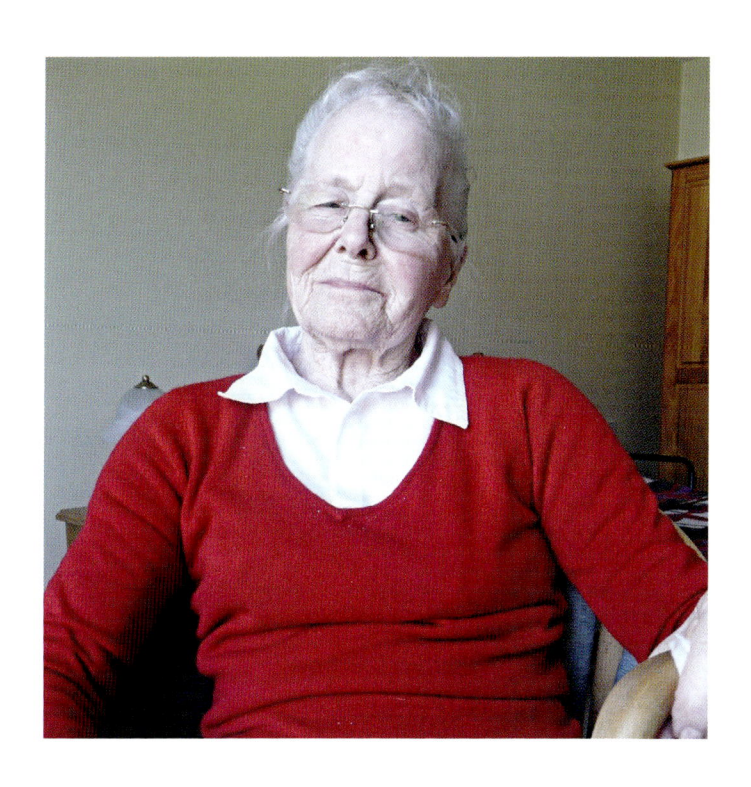

'I prefer to be downstairs and not in my room because I like company. I enjoy listening to the music although I am not musical myself. I am not a very sociable person. I like to be near people but I like to be on the outside of things.'

Joan Wade

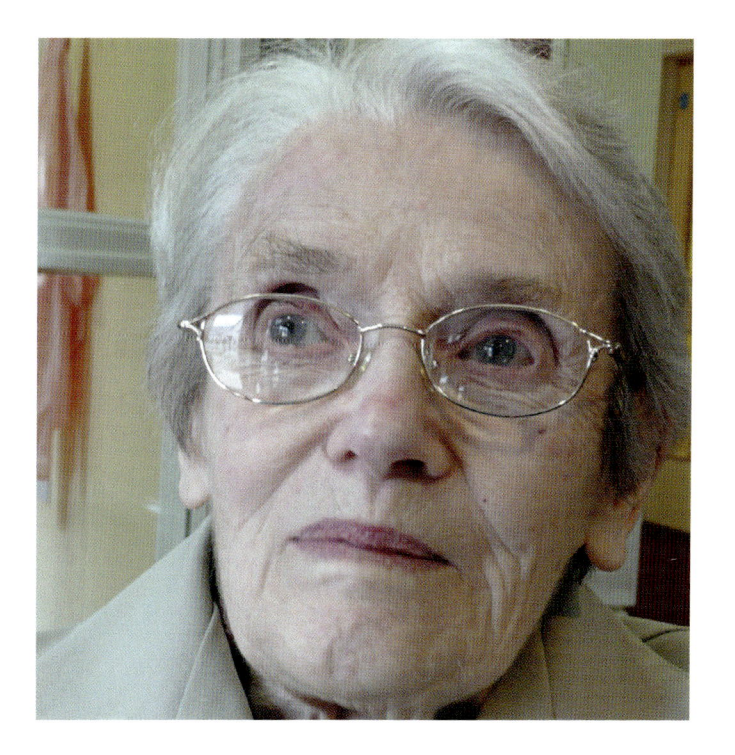

Mary Cave loves talking to people.
'I came here because I coudn't look after myself. I became very forgetful. I used to be a nanny. I loved looking after babies. I took over after the monthly nurse. Now the children have children of their own.'

Rosemary soon made her space, her place and her home.

'This is home to me.

For two years I came here for day care and respite care. Moving in here was not a problem for me, it was like coming home. ***It was a great relief for my family to know that I was safe.*** *When your house has been your home for fifty years it is hard to give it up but I couldn't manage the stairs so it was not viable to be at home.*

When I am in my room I like to have the door open. I like to see what is going on and I like hearing voices. I love reading, doing crossword puzzles and I have started watching television since I have been here.

I have always been a "joiner"; I belonged to groups such as the Women's Institute, Bowls Club, the Civic Trust and the Mothers Union. I've had years of going out and about so I am thankful for what I have had. It is not so easy for me to get about now using a wheelchair and minibus. But life is what you make it.'

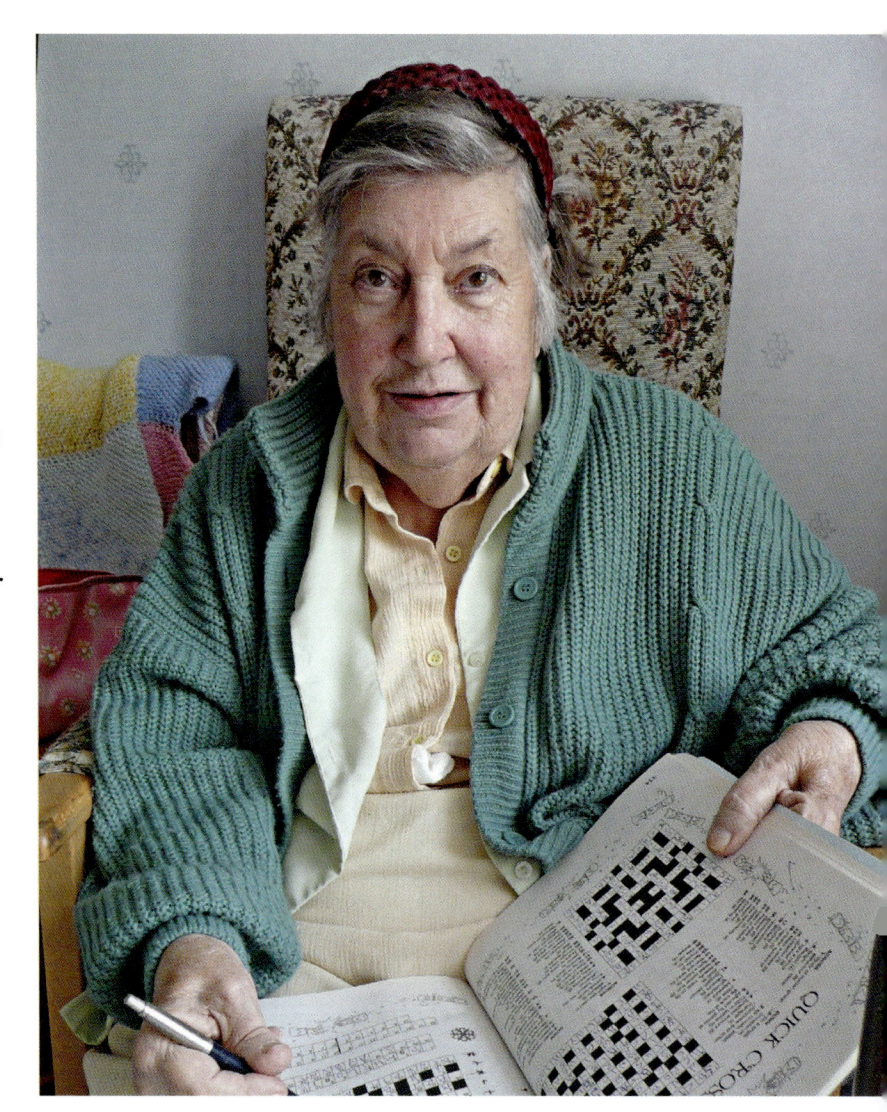

Rosemary is well known in Malmesbury for making lace.

'I loved school and won a County Scholarship to Malmesbury School before I was eleven. I was the youngest girl in the whole school. I was there until I was sixteen and was a prefect for one term. I left school with the School Certificate in seven subjects. I went to work on the Post Office counter in Malmesbury and married a postman. He had his eye on me since I was thirteen. He was a telegram boy, wore a uniform with a little round hat and rode a bicycle. He did his National Service before we married. **Before he went he was the spottiest boy you ever saw but when he came back he was gorgeous, so dishy. Wow! We married when I was twenty two, and all my wedding clothes were borrowed.**

I had always wanted to make lace.

I met Doreen Campbell who showed me her lace and that started me off. I used to travel with her all over the country to lace making days. Each time I went I bought more patterns, threads and bobbins.

My masterpiece is the lace edging for the altar cloth for Brokenborough Church. I made it as a gift. It was worked in Gutterman silk and was made up of fifty two repeats of the pattern and each one took three hours.'

A section of the lace edging from the altar cloth in St. John the Baptist Church, Brokenborough.

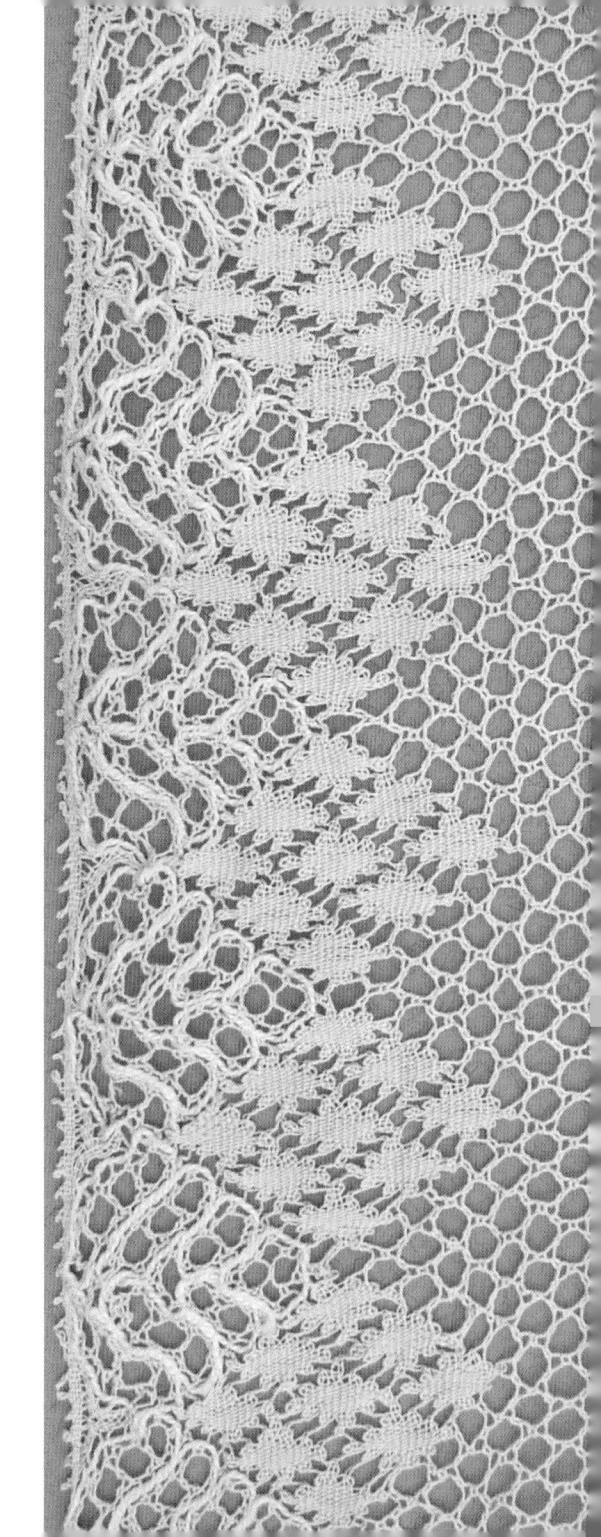

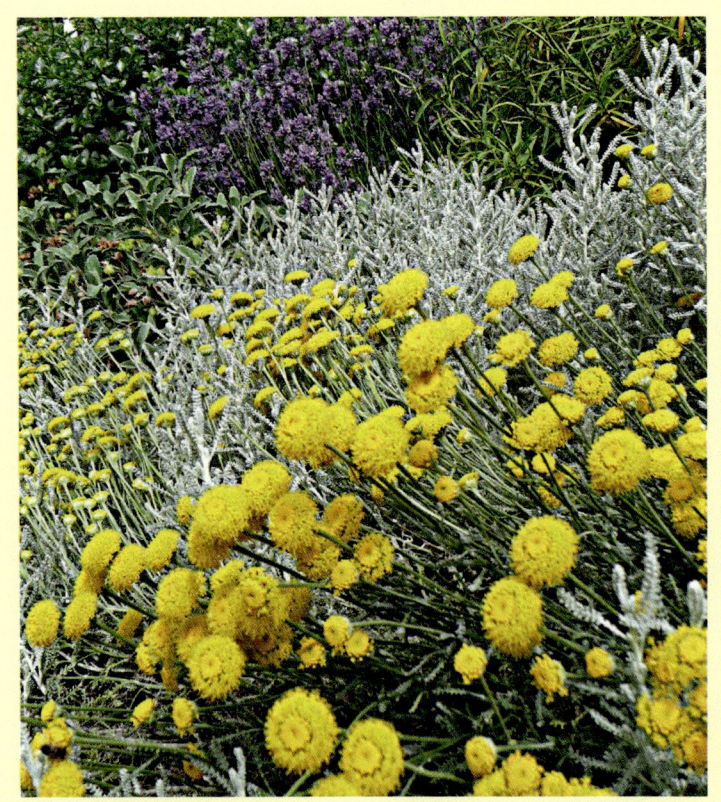

'I loved gardening. I was a flower gardener. My daughter says that I was a real expert.'

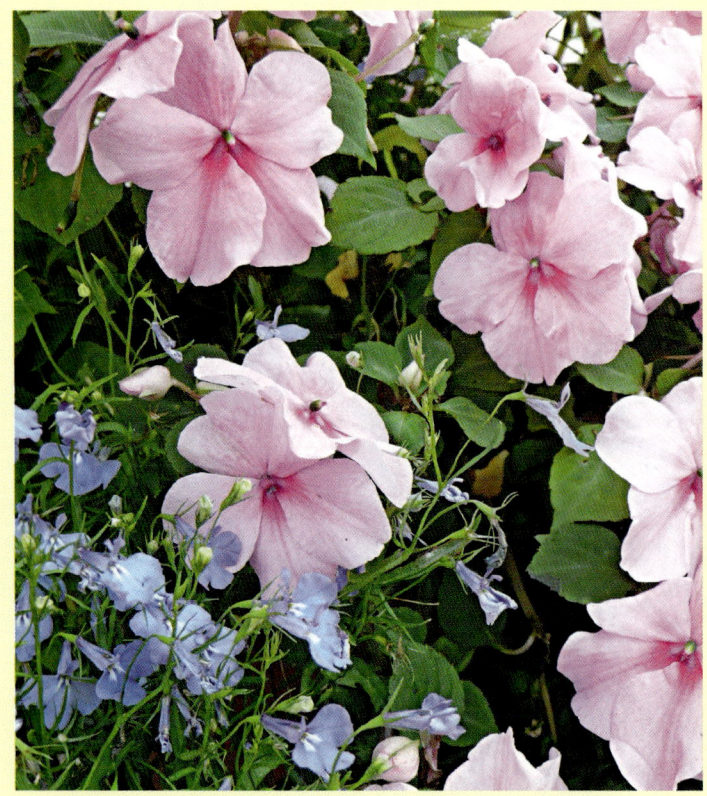

Hetty

'I loved my garden. I was working in the garden all the time.'

Dorothy

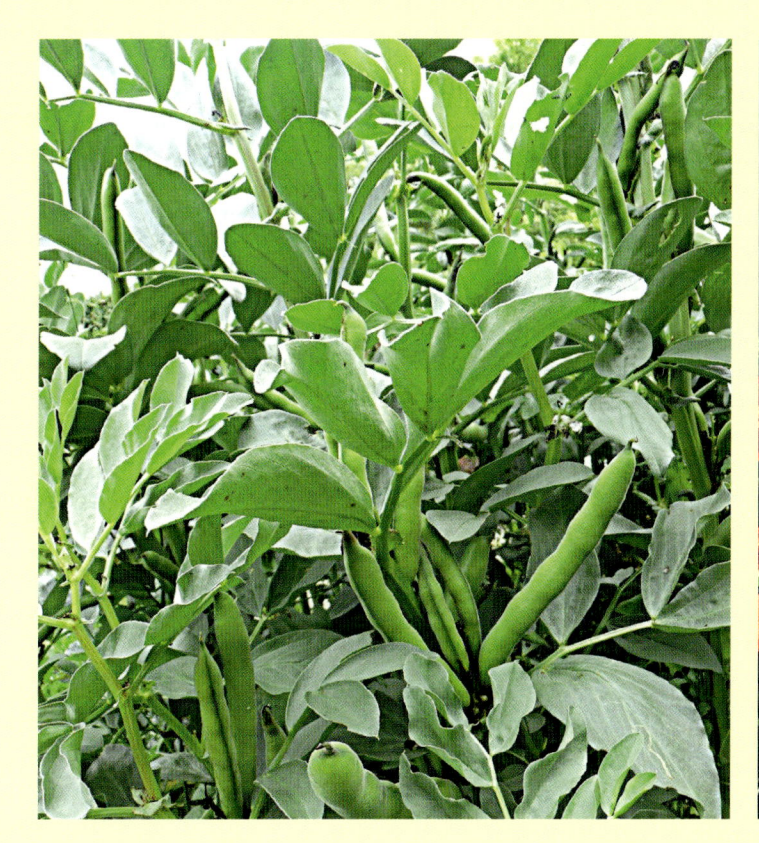

'When I had a place of my own I loved gardening.'

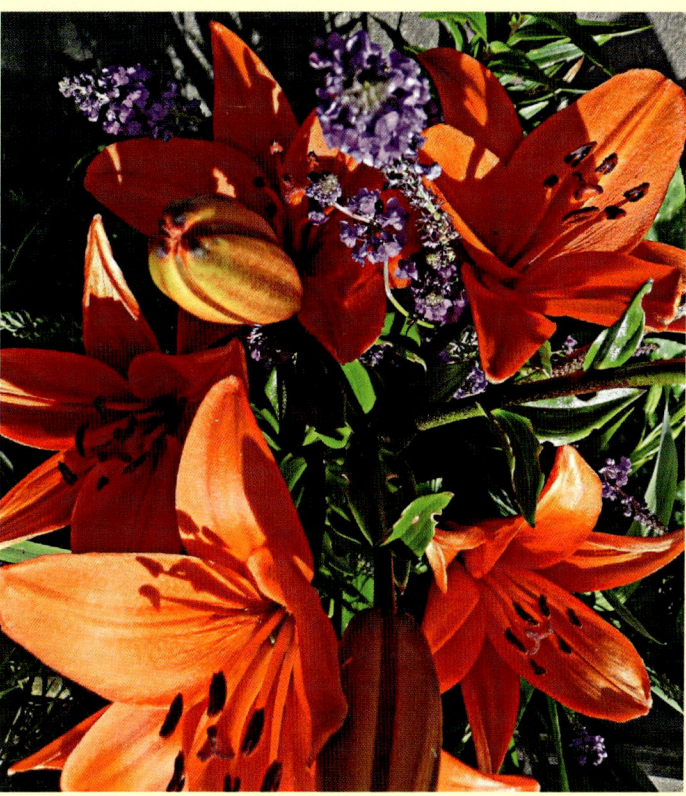

Lottie

'I was a great gardener. It takes the worries away being with the flowers and the bees, how hard they work. I miss my garden.'

Queenie

Jesse used to live in Oaksey.

'There I won the Best Kept Garden in the village for four years and I won the North Wiltshire District Council Best Kept Garden for two years.

The garden was overgrown when I moved there. It was hard to clear it to make the lawns, flower beds and vegetable garden. I took photographs of my garden as I went along. I grew roses and a friend said to me, **"Look at those roses. Look at the colours. How have you got them to go together like that?"** I told him that I didn't plan them, I just looked for a space then planted another rose!
I've enjoyed my life, I really have.'
Jesse Baldock

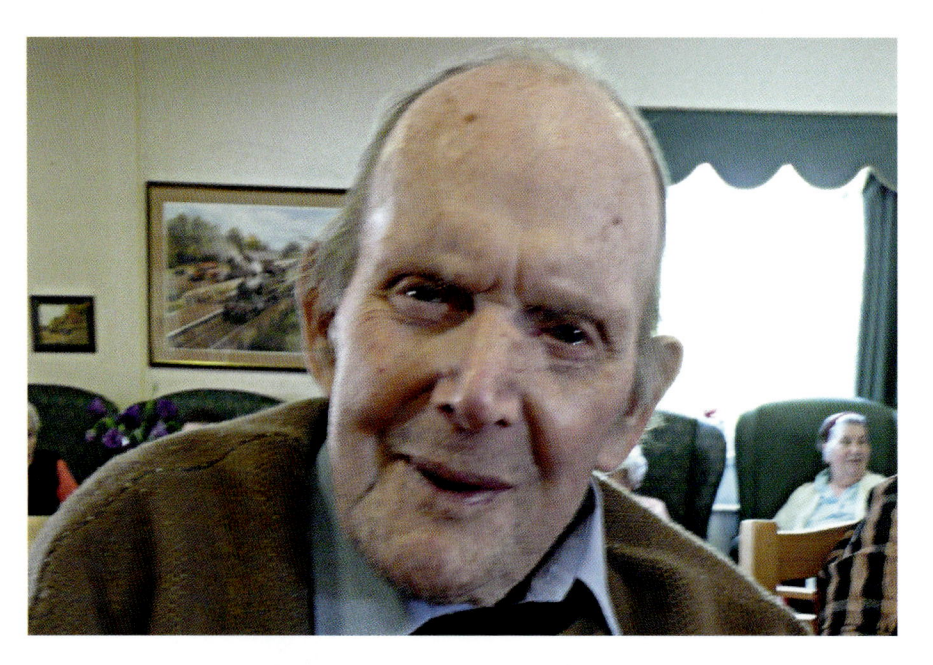

Jesse was born in 1910. He worked on the same farm for forty years.

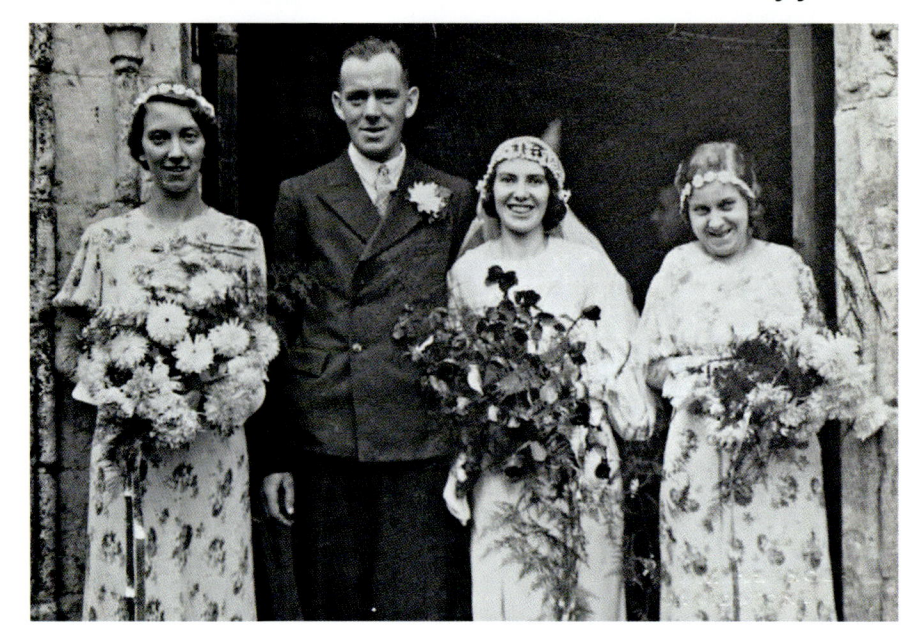

Jesse married Carol in 1936. *'Carol was six years younger than me.'*

63

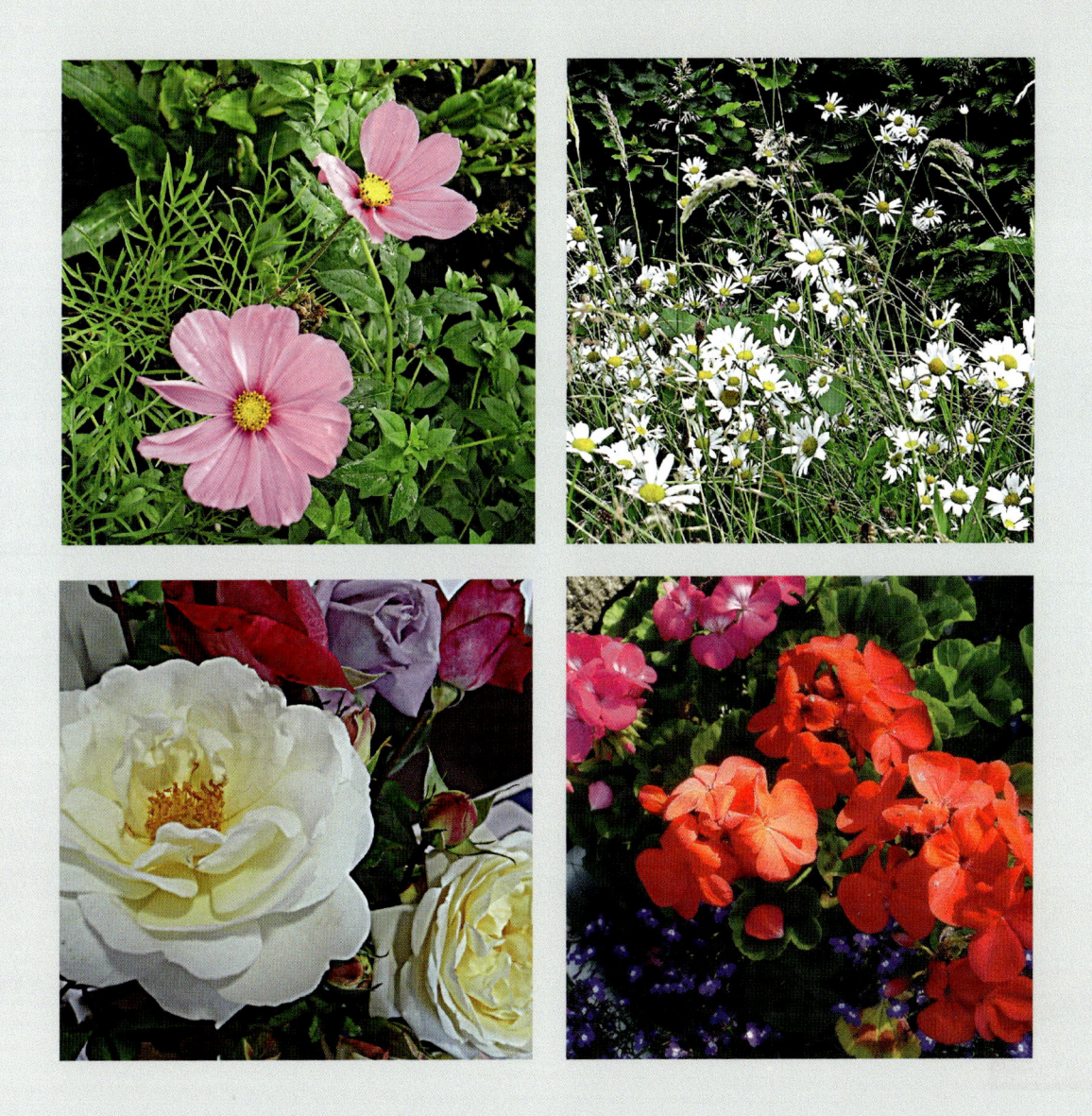

The Courtyard

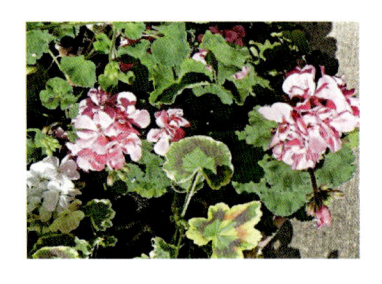

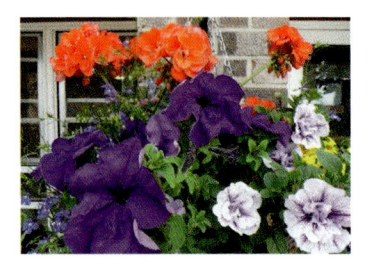

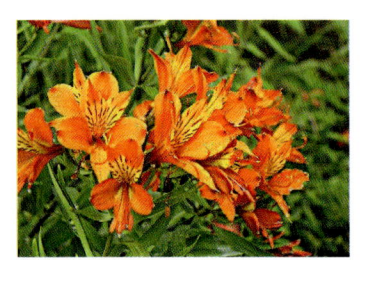

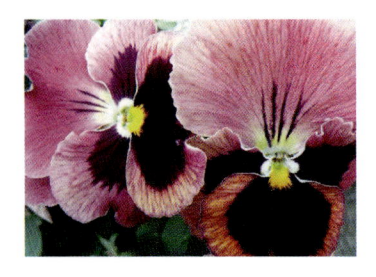

I sit in the courtyard in the warm summer sun,
Surrounded by blooms, competitions they've won.
The colours dance gracefully in the breeze,
Rustling around are one or two leaves.
Standing proud are the sunflower heads
Shadowing the pansies below in their beds.
Tubs overflow with petal and stem
More are all ready to replace them.
Hanging baskets, flourish plants.
Plants tumble and fall
While others sweep eagerly
Across a once plain wall.
As I sit with a smile upon my face
My memories I share with this beautiful place.

Bill Muir

Bill's love of plants comes from his career as an Estate Manager in Surrey where he lived with his wife, Jessie, for fifty years.

Ill health forced Bill to make his home in Burnham House.

'It's like a marriage, a gamble that you hope will work out well. I like my own company but I can have company when I want it. It is an asset when life becomes much slower. **People talk to you here.** *I am glad not to be on my own in my own home because I wouldn't have the energy for my six grandchildren and two great grandchildren. I like reading and definitely do not watch a lot of television, I am very selective. Documentaries interest me and I really enjoy the wildlife programmes.*

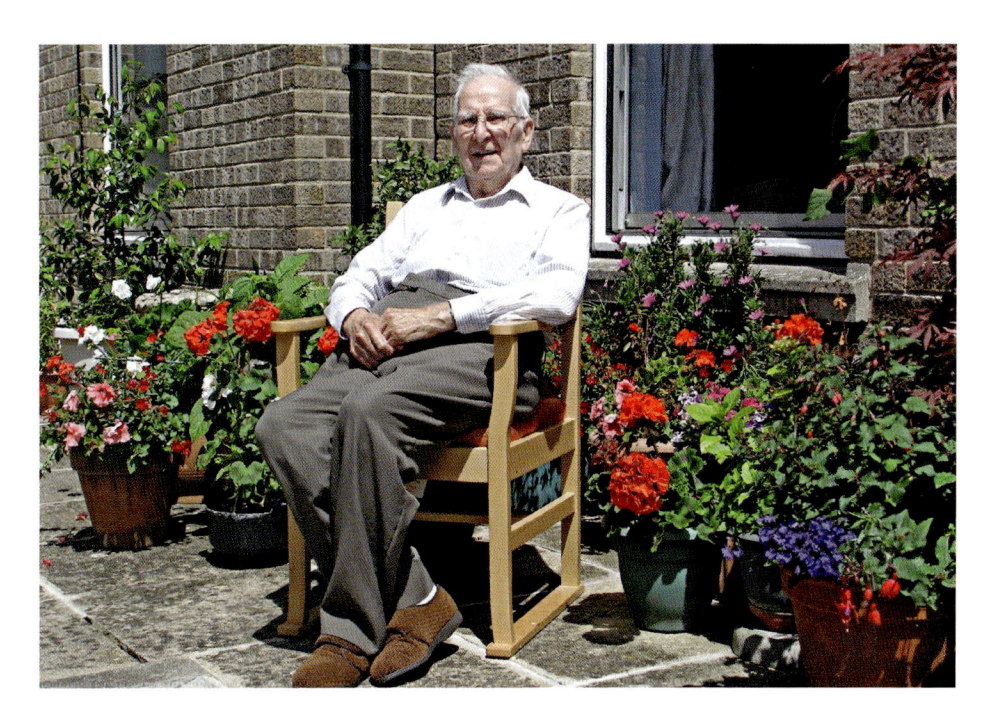

'I sit in the Courtyard in the warm summer sun...'

I met my wife when I was posted to Oxford during the war. Jessie was working in a munitions factory and I was in the Army. We were married for sixty three years. In marriage it is important to understand each other's problems and to both pull on the same end of the rope, not against each other.

Life is hard and disappointing at times but to have faith in what you are doing comes from experience.

During the war I was an Army Instructor training raw recruits. My posting was to prepare for invasion. Training was basically how to kill without getting killed yourself.'

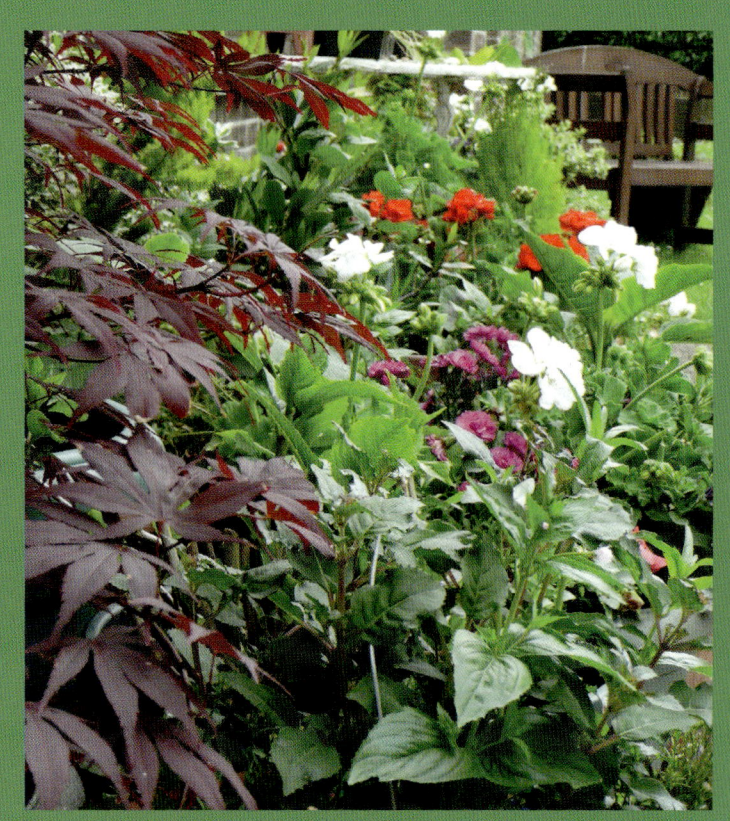

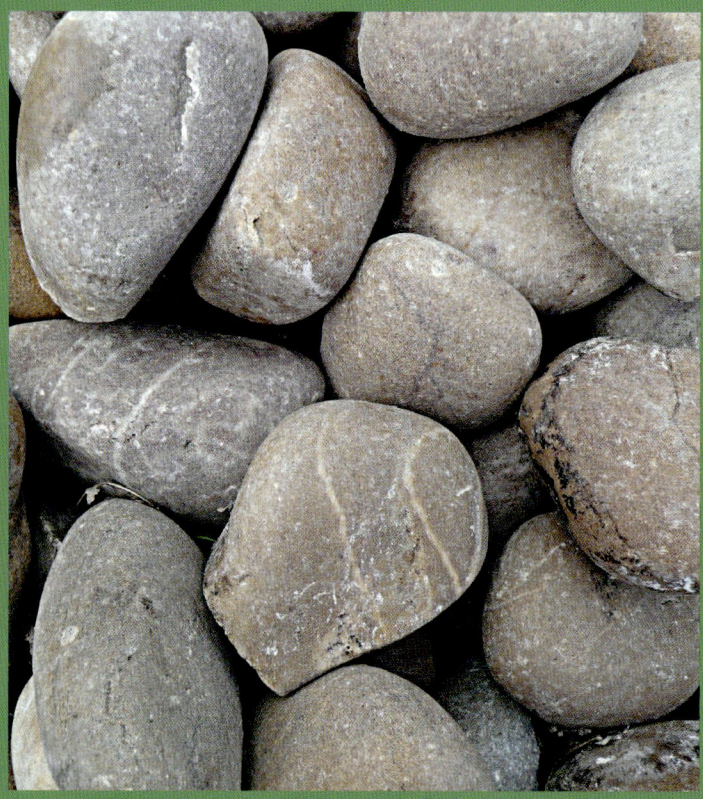

The Burnham House garden is a lovely place... **to watch the birds bathing in the fountain...**

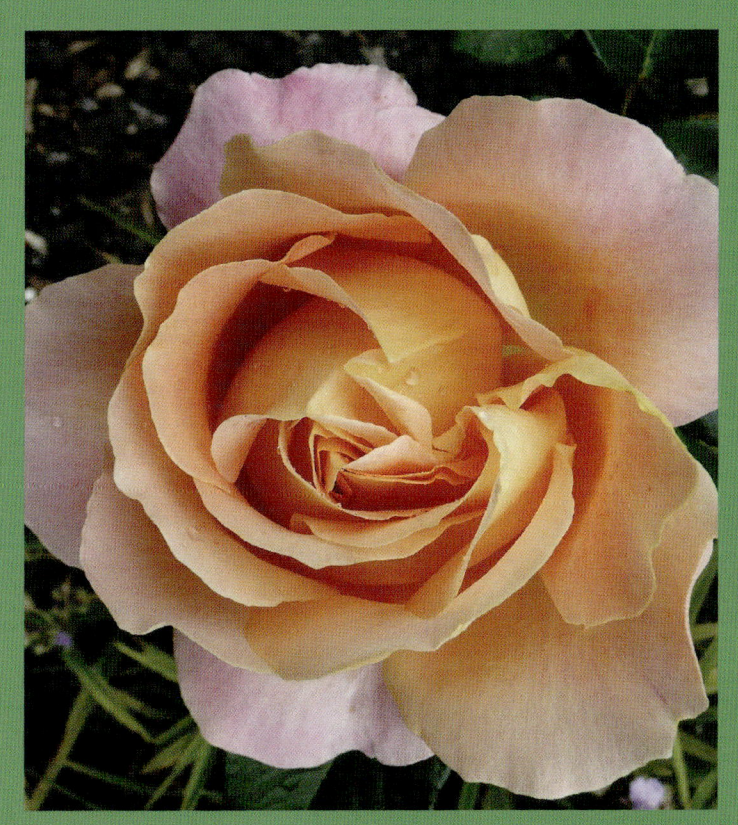

to chat with friends and family...

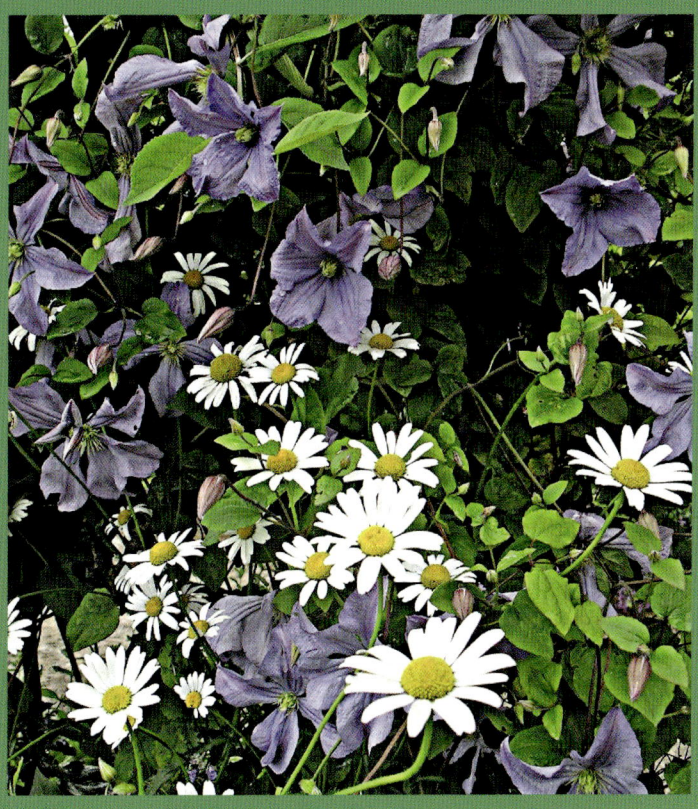

to enjoy a cream tea or an ice cream.

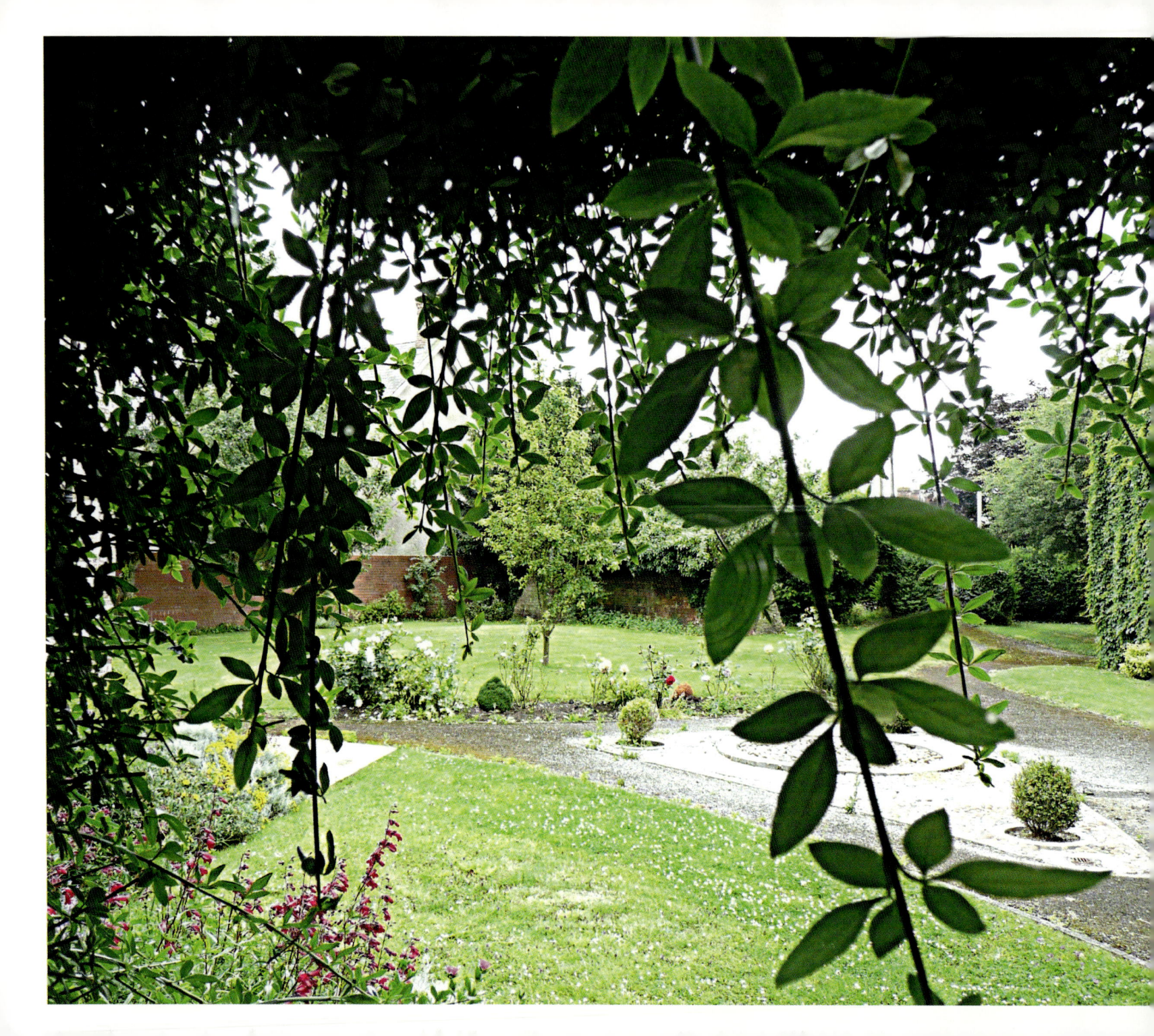

Farewell to Burnham House - 2 July 2008

'Burnham House first opened as a Day Centre in 1977,' recalls Day Centre Manager, Daphne White.

'The Mayor and several local organisations raised money for furniture and equipment for the house and pupils from Corn Gastons School decorated the rooms.

I started to work here as the Cook in 1980 when new accommodation was built next to the original house. The building opened with invitations to the public to see the facilities provided by the Rural District Council and Wiltshire County Council. There were fifty bedrooms, a dining room and sitting rooms to accommodate the residents and the twenty Day Centre places for care from Monday to Friday.

In 1986 I applied for the position of Care Officer and was pleased to be appointed because I had always enjoyed helping the residents.

In 2000 Wiltshire County Council transferred the management of the home to The Orders of St. John Care Trust and a year later I took over running the Day Centre.

When "The Friends of Burnham House" was launched it was a model for other homes. The "Friends" supported the Home, raised funds and contributed to installing the garden fountain.

I really enjoy helping people to take part in the inter-house activities and gardening or flower competitions. We have won some of them.'

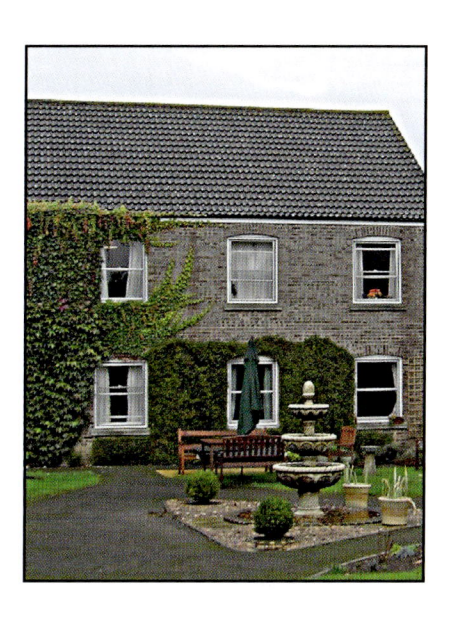

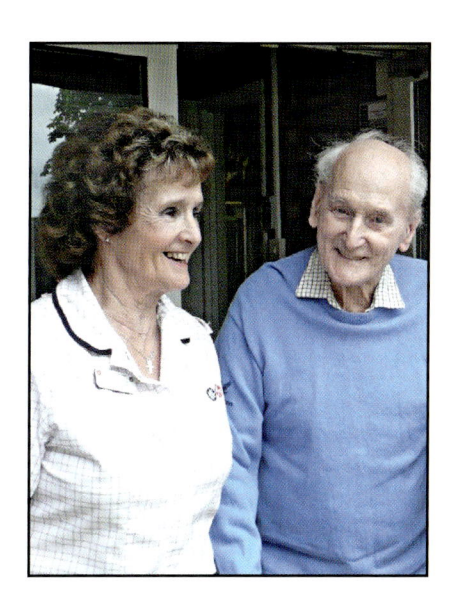

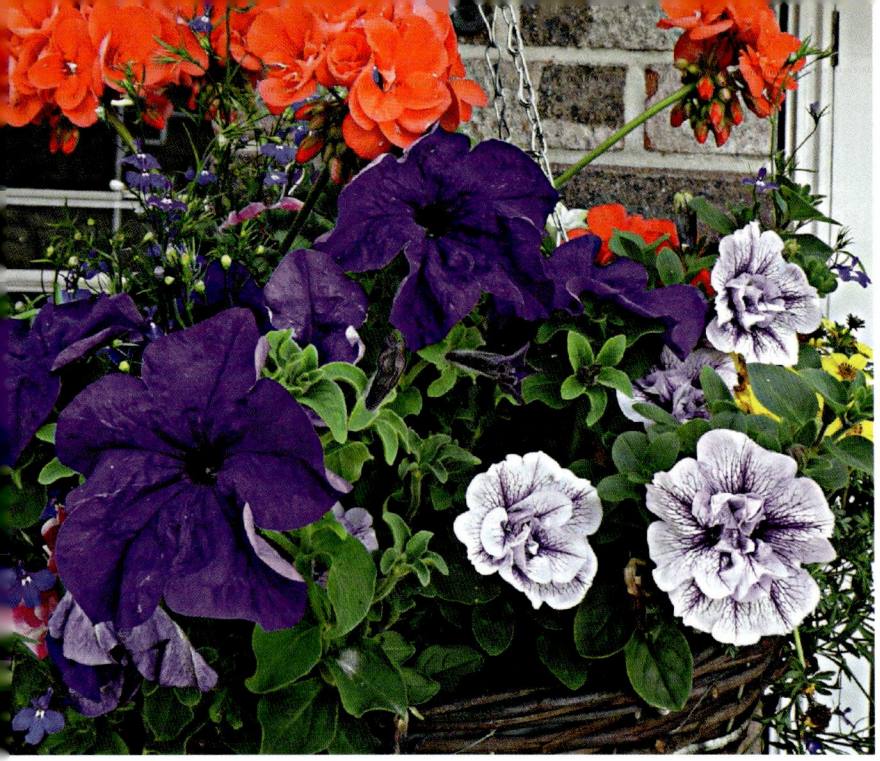

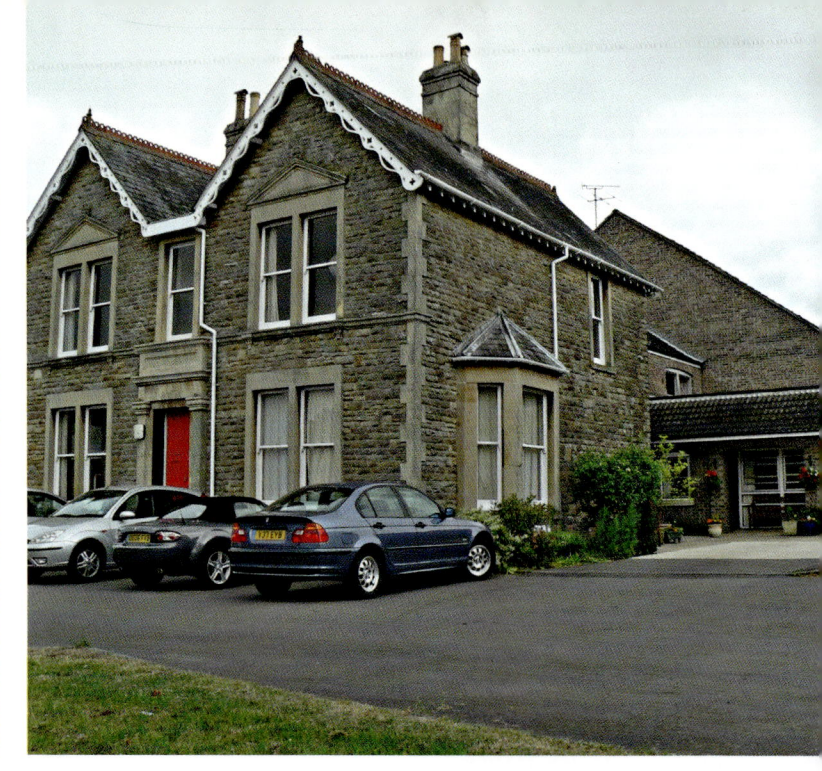

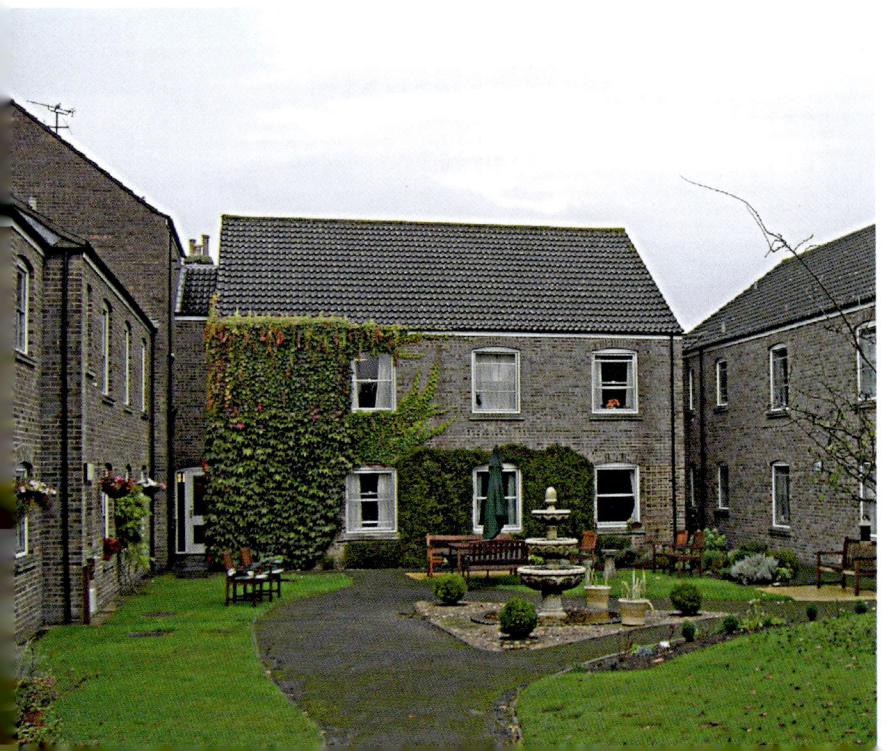

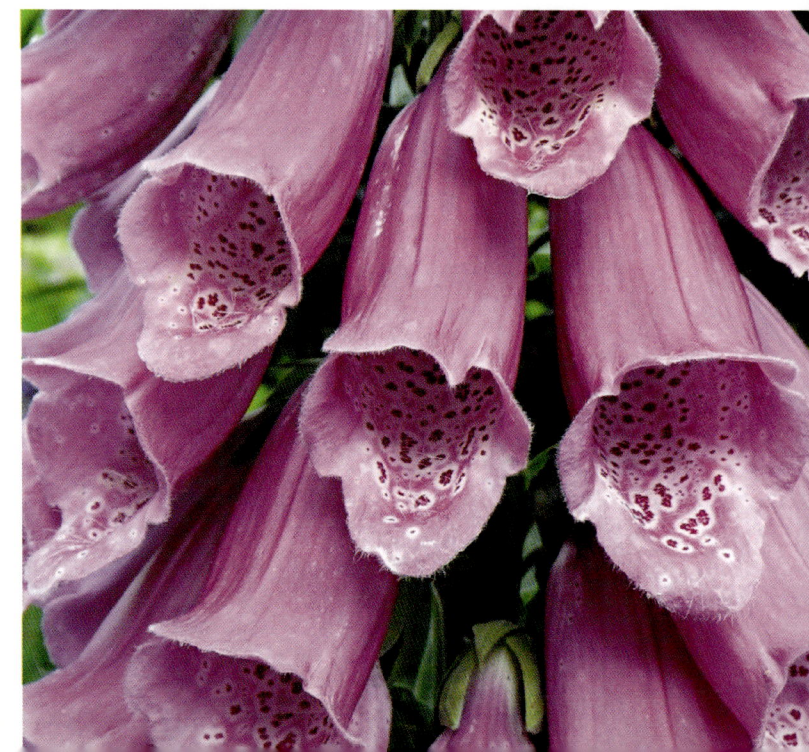

Acknowledgements

I am indebted to the residents of Burnham House who patiently and willingly shared their time and experiences with me.
Also I wish to acknowledge the interest and help given to me by their families and friends.

I am grateful to the staff at Burnham House and Athelstan House for their support and in particular to:
Home Manager, Burnham House, Elaine Andrews
Home Manager, Athelstan House, Charlotte Sievewright
Activities Manager, Martin Spalding and Assistant, Trish Warren
Day Centre Manager, Daphne White
Day Centre Carer, Estella King

I appreciate the support received from:
Wiltshire County Director, The Orders of St. John Care Trust, Diane Bowden

North Wiltshire District Council's Malmesbury Area Committee

Wiltshire County Council

Burnham House Arts Project Evaluator: Julie Brandstatter and my proof readers.

Acknowledgement of photographs provided by
The Orders of St. John Care Trust and staff at Burnham House: pages 28 (Left), 41, 51 (Left), 65 and the two exterior views of Burnham House.

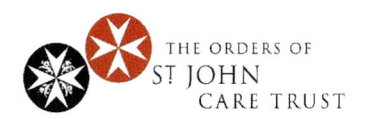

THE ORDERS OF ST JOHN CARE TRUST

blurb

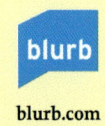

blurb.com